The Dawn of the Health Age

'HE DAWN OF THE HEALTH AGE

" Lift up your eyes, and look on the fields ; for th
are white already to harvest."

THE DAWN OF THE HEALTH AGE

BY

BENJAMIN MOORE

M.A., D.Sc., M.R.C.S., L.R.C.P.

23307

LONDON

J. & A. CHURCHILL

7 GT. MARLBOROUGH ST.

LIVERPOOL

THE LIVERPOOL BOOKSELLERS'
CO. LTD.

70 LORD STREET

1911

Printed by BALLANTYNE, HANSON & Co.
At the Ballantyne Press, Edinburgh

PREFACE

THIS book is intended to demonstrate, on clear, broad lines, the necessity for entirely remodelling the present system of medical service in the interests of the whole community.

It shows that hundreds of thousands of lives and millions of money can be saved every year if disease is attacked on scientific principles, instead of being dallied with as at present.

It proves that such a course is best both for the millionaire and the pauper, because there is but one set of disease agents in the whole world, which attack rich and poor alike, and are transmitted from the one to the other.

There is not one word of party politics in the book from cover to cover, and readers and reviewers are requested to attach no *labels* to it, but to judge it honestly on its own merits.

In the interests of our common humanity, and to aid in the evolution of a fitter and healthier race, it is addressed equally to conservative and liberal, to humanitarian and economist, to capitalist and labourist, to individualist and socialist.

All the great political parties in our State are

committed by public utterances of their leaders,
and by the tide of public opinion, to social
reform, and the hygienic aspect of social reform
is the most dominant of all, commanding the
whole situation.

Poverty and destitution simply cannot exist
amongst a fit, virile, healthy nation. Banish
acute and chronic infectious diseases, teach
temperate and normal habits of eating, drinking, and living, making the reverse a crime, and
poverty and suffering in corresponding measure
must decrease.

The passion for drugging and doctoring the
individual with specific cures and quack nostrums
is one of the prepotent curses of our time;
while the health and well-being of the species,
and all things making for fitness of the race,
are neglected.

We allow diseases to invade and enfeeble us,
then ruin our systems with drugs in attempting
to exorcise the demon of disease, and when we
fail we turn to the claptrap of faith-healing or
homœopathy, imbued with all the spirit of the
superstition and idolatry of the Middle Ages.

Take up any daily paper or monthly maga-
zine and look at the columns and pages of
costly advertisements devoted to quack medicines and remedies of all kinds, reflect on the
thousands of pounds spent by poor human gulls
in supporting these frauds and the authors of
them, and then ask yourself, is it not nearly
time that we had some rational system of dealing

with disease and protecting people from their own ignorance?

It is only a strong public feeling, demanding a rationally constituted public medical service armed with powers to fight disease, which can bring reform in these matters.

BENJAMIN MOORE.

Shrewsbury Road,
  Birkenhead, *Oct.* 1910.

CONTENTS

THE DAWN OF THE
HEALTH AGE

CHAPTER I

2 3 3 0 7

HOW WE TINKER WITH DISEASE INSTEAD OF STOPPING IT

At the present moment we possess sufficient knowledge of medical science to enable us to save at least three hundred thousand lives every year in this country alone, and the saving of these three hundred thousand valuable lives could all be effected without costing the nation a single penny, but rather at the same time many million pounds a year might be saved which under present conditions are absolutely wasted.

In the face of all this spendthrift extravagance in lives and money, we eagerly call for more scientific research to enable us to cope with disease, utterly ignoring the rich harvest which medical science has already yielded ready to be garnered all around us.

It is true that we are still ignorant of the causes and modes of propagation of certain diseases, and attempts to discover these are in

A

themselves most laudable; but it is equally true, and much more important, that we do know perfectly well how to combat some of the direst and most common diseases, and that we move neither hand nor foot to do so, but stand benumbed and useless, as if we were a race of savages without any polity or system of government or capacity for any concerted plan of action for the national welfare.

The problems of disease, from which radically spring all the most important problems of social reform, require now to be tackled by statesmen, and not by doctors and scientists.

The exponents of medical science have accomplished their aims in many important directions and have laid their results before the public; they can proceed no further without concerted statesmanlike action, and it is for the public now to awaken statesmen into activity.

While a statesman can to a certain extent give definiteness and objective to reform, he alone cannot move unless the public are ready for the forward movement.

There are signs present even now of awakening interest of the public in health problems, as shown by the general approval of foreshadowed legislation dealing with some of the great problems of social reform, commencing with invalidity insurance and reform of the Poor Law, especially on the medical aspect which furnishes the key to the whole situation.

It is method more than money that we want in order to combat and conquer in our battles with disease; we must fight in the future by means of a disciplined army instead of, as at present, with an undisciplined mob, each member doing what is right in his own eyes and working at cross purposes to his neighbour.

It is not the slightest exaggeration to say that our present methods of attacking disease are mediæval in their antiquity and their ignorance.

The scheme which is here to be laid down is most benevolent and most charitable, both to those now afflicted with disease and those of all ranks of society which it proposes to save from the clutches of disease and untimely death; but attention is asked for it not primarily on benevolent or charitable grounds, but mainly as an economic scheme that will save millions of pounds annually to the nation.

All misdirected labour is labour wasted, and the labour of the thirty-two thousand medical men at present practising in this country is almost wasted as far as the health of the community which they serve is concerned. Anything more futile, less scientific, more hopelessly absurd than the present method of dealing with disease can scarcely be conceived. Constant association has blinded us to this topsy-turvy want of all system and all method in tackling disease problems which has slumbered on in our midst from generation to generation in despite of all our advance in knowledge of medical science.

With a self-satisfied air we make survey of what we term the modern advances in medicine and surgery, *as applied to tinkering the diseased individual,* and complacently the credulous public swallows the glorification, while we slumber over the thousand-fold greater achievements possible to organised effort in the wholesale eradication of disease from the commonwealth. Meanwhile hundreds of thousands of the fittest of our citizens die yearly without one effort being made to save them.

Naturally our organised army of doctors would have to be paid, and this would cost the nation eight to ten millions a year; but this money is all paid now, and more than paid. All that is necessary is to pay it through different channels, and the advantage gained is that we shall possess, as aforesaid, an army instead of a mob.

Needless to say, no disrespect is meant to the medical profession by designating it as a mob. That term is only intended to signify that it is entirely lacking in the first elements of organisation so far as dealing with the diseases of the nation is concerned, and preserving the nation in a fit state of health.

There is no more noble profession than that of medicine; it is one which is only too sacrificing of its own interests; there is no profession which does so much for charity without recompense sought or obtained. Charitable work is the bane and curse of the medical profession, as it is of the nation at large, and the constant exploitation of doctors by hospitals and Poor Law municipal agencies is a disgrace to our times.

But speaking of the medical profession as a whole, it is developed upon wrong and anti-quated lines of tinkering the individual for fees after he has fallen into ill-health, and it is impossible for it from within to organise itself into an army of health and public safety against disease, which shall seek disease at its source and commence to deal with this large problem of eradication in a modern and scientific way.

Even if it set about reorganising itself on new lines, the profession lacks those effective com-pulsory powers of dealing with disease which will be elaborated in subsequent chapters, and these only can be given to it by legislation.

The problem of saving these hundreds of thousands of lives and millions of pounds of money annually is accordingly one for the public itself, led by those publicists who take an interest in medico-social problems.

It cannot be too strongly reiterated in this introductory chapter that what is required for the successful solution of this gigantic problem is method, method, and once again method. In the first place, we must form our highly organised and equipped Army of Health; and, in the second place, we must give that army plenary powers by legislation to deal with disease on the lines which scientific research has disclosed for us in the past generation.

This plenary power to fight disease will not in the slightest degree prejudice the rights of the individual sufferer from disease, but, on the contrary, will give him double the chance of recovery, while at the same time it will protect the healthy from the danger of infection.

Under the new regime, medical treatment will be as free to every one as is the school and education to-day, and every one must accept medical treatment in his own interest and that of the community, just as he must to-day accept education for his child, whether he wants to or not.

After ten years of such a system, nine-tenths of the disease and almost an equal proportion of the destitution will be found no longer amidst our population, and the benefit will be felt not only amongst the working classes, but from palace to hovel—if indeed hovels still exist.

The Briton, in the opinion of some superficial critics, will become a slave under such compulsory conditions when his home—his castle of dirt, ignorance, and disease—is visited by the health officer, and so he is advised to fight to the last gasp against such inspection. But there is, fortunately, also a clean Briton, an educated Briton, a hard-working Briton ; he exists already by the hundred thousand amongst t', working classes, and he is rapidly becom'nt a power in the land. This type of Briton is acquiring new and strange ideas of liberty; strange to say, he believes in education, and has no objection to his indolent and ignorant neighbour being punished for neglecting to send his children to school. The school officer is not to his mind a tool of the Holy Inquisition; and, similarly, he has only to realise that he and his wife and children stand in danger, in real mortal danger, of being infected and destroyed by the disease harboured by the filth and ignorance next door, in order to let the health officer attack and remove that filth and disease. When thoroughly awakened by the new preachers of health, the virile, healthy type of Briton may be depended upon to be so anxious for the health of body of himself and those near and dear to him that no power on earth will long prevent the necessary legislation, and reform will come with the ever-growing velocity of an avalanche. Our new health army may be an inquisition, but what an inquisition it is—one of knowledge against ignorance, of health against disease, of life against death, of salvation against damnation.

Who would not welcome such an inquisition? If this be slavery, let us welcome our chains, and be bondsmen in a cause such as the world has never seen. Here is a crusade worth joining, a fight worth waging, a fight that can be won—nay, a fight that must be won. For more rapid success we must, however,

win to our cause the cautious and stolid economist, and so, in concluding this introduction, let
us show what vast stores of gold, which being
transmuted means energy and work done, can
be saved and accumulated every year through
the operations of this Army of Health; let us
point out the spoils of this bloodless warfare.

It has been stated above that we already pay
for the health army, but not in such a manner
that we can either organise it or set it to fight.
These payments that we already make, and
which collectively give the doctors their none
too magnificent livings, are now so exacted in
fees, varying according to our incomes, the rich
man paying a bigger and the poor man a smaller
fee, that there would be but little variation if
the sum were raised by taxation; and so this
taxation would mean no additional drain on
the nation, for we would not then have to pay
the doctors their fees privately and directly,
but would have full and free treatment when
we needed it. Of course, disease would in a
few years become so abated that the treatment
aspect would be at a minimum; we should,
fortunately for us, rarely need treatment, and
nearly all the work would be work of inspection, instruction on how to live healthily, and
prevention of the incidence of disease by pounc-
ing on every infectious case and isolating it at
once. Still, as far as disease did still exist, the
State Health Army doctor would attend to it.
Accordingly, apart from some initial expense

for hospitals and sanatoria—necessary until the army of consumptives, for example, had been reduced from its present figure of about one hundred and fifty thousand of unfortunate sufferers travelling to a certain death, to less, say, than five hundred throughout the whole country—apart from this initial expense, no fresh money is required for the scheme, but only a new organisation, and a payment of our doctors' fees as a tax to Government, instead of directly to the private doctor.

Now, let us look at the other side of the balance-sheet, and leaving out all question of lives saved and the happiness that accompanies better health, let us pay attention to pounds sterling alone.

The magnitude of the Annual Disease Budget which ill-health, consequent loss of employment, destitution of widows and children consequent upon illness, and later the death of fathers from preventable disease, costs the nation is undoubtedly colossal, but difficult of accurate estimation. It can be stated with considerable probability to be located somewhere about one hundred million pounds annually. This is a truly colossal sum; one poor half-year of it, if it could be raised in any way and applied to clear away the causes of disease, would be more than sufficient to stop the whole hideous panorama of disease and destitution; but, alas! we are in the grip of a vicious circle.

One has only to spend a few minutes in

reflecting upon how disease does its work of destruction, to see how the millions mount up.

If we take that biggest scourge of all diseases, viz. tuberculosis, as an example, we have in Great Britain and Ireland about 150,000 affected individuals at one time. We may take it that the disease runs an average course of two years before the curtain is drawn, and as it is a disease occurring at all ages, it is probable that of the 150,000 sufferers, two-thirds, or 100,000, are adults capable of employment. As a result of the disease, not only the sufferers, but their families and dependents if they have any, are thrown on the support of others. All the time, it must be remembered, these 150,000 are infecting others, while we do nothing to prevent the process, so that the horrible tale is made perpetual, and the economic loss goes on year after year. Since consumption is considerably commoner nowadays amongst men than amongst women, we may take it that of the 150,000 of the army of tuberculosis at least 60,000 are adult males; and if these be taken at the low average wage of one pound sterling a week, the annual loss of wages alone is a sum of £3,000,000, to which we may certainly add another £1,000,000 for lost female labour, making £4,000,000 for wages alone. Of the 150,000 sufferers, about 75,000 die every year, and the melancholy item of funeral expenses must cost a sum worth saving. At least one-third of these poor unfortunates die in Poor Law or other public institutions ; [1] but wherever they die, the expense falls ultimately on the nation, for any expense broadly enough distributed amongst some hundreds of thousands of people becomes indistinguishable from a national expense.   Each individual upon whom it falls, sinking down, pulls upon others all around him to help him in his calamity, and ultimately the burden of phthisis, just as it is propagated and carried to us all, rich or poor, by the same common microbe, falls to be borne as to its finance in the same common way by the whole community. In nine-tenths of the cases, sooner or later it comes on the rates, just as do insanity, alcoholism, and all other forms of long-continued or chronic disease.

But the actual wages lost in the period of illness of the phthisical patient, considerable as we have just seen it to be, is insignificant compared to the burden of destitution left as its aftermath, first upon the family survivors and later on the community.

The widows and orphans fall nearly always to the State or community to maintain, and, alas ! history will have a sad tale to tell as to how we have, up till now, been looking after these

[1] The cost of tubercular patients to the Poor Law Institutions is at least one and a half millions a year; those belonging to Friendly Societies and in Sick Benefit cost their Societies over one million a year ; and Voluntary Charities and Sanatoria for the Consumptive cost almost half a million.   In addition we have over 100,000 cripples with decreased earning powers, and about eighty per cent. of these owe their lameness to tubercular disease.

unfortunate orphans and turning them into un-
desirables in the General Mixed Workhouses, or
in immoral and dissolute homes.[1]

We are, however, just now dealing with
economics, and so may attempt to get at some
idea of how much the widows and orphans of
deceased phthisical fathers cost the nation.
The estimate is most difficult. In some cases
the adult dying from phthisis happily leaves no
children behind; in other cases three or four
are left to be brought up by the parish for
periods varying from ten years downwards; but
if it be taken that it averages out at one child
to be maintained, schooled, clothed, and fed for
ten years, this, at a cost of only four shillings a
week, works out at £10 a year, or £100 for the
ten years. If we take the modest estimate that
there are 30,000 deaths a year in the United
Kingdom necessitating such provision, the sum
of £3,000,000 a year is obtained. If we add
this orphans' maintenance to wages loss, we
have a sum of at least seven million pounds.

We have as yet by no means exhausted the
financial drain on the nation due to tuberculosis,
for economically this is the most expensive of
all diseases upon the community. This arises
from the fact that, on account of its modes of
propagation, pulmonary phthisis takes off most
of its victims between the ages of twenty-five
and forty-five years, just when economically they
are of the highest value to the community, in the

[1] See Reports of Royal Commission on Poor Law.

nidst of their best working and wage-earning
oower.

Not only do we lose the wages of each
ohthisical workman during the later part of
nis period of illness, when, on an average, as
statistics show, he takes more than a full year's
sick benefit out of his society; and not only
nave we to support in our poorhouses his orphan
children after he has gone; in addition, the
community as a whole suffers from the loss of
nany years of the services and work done by
he workman which would have accrued had
consumption not cut him off in his prime. The
average age has been shown to be only forty
years at which phthisical workmen are removed,
whereas in the absence of phthisis, and with
heir expectations of life at the age at which
ohthisis fell upon them, they would have lived
and worked on the average to fifty-five years.
t follows that while we only gain economically
oy the death to the extent of the food, cloth-
ng, and other wants actually consumed by the
workman himself, and spared by his death, we
ose economically the fifteen years' labour, re-
oresented by fifteen years' wages, which the
workman would have turned out had phthisis
not seized him. On an average this loss may
oe set down at least at £20 a year—probably it
would be more—and this multiplied by fifteen,
or the fifteen years, gives the national value of
each of these workmen cut off at forty, instead
of fifty-five, at £300. If, on this basis, we take

it that of the 75,000 deaths annually in the
United Kingdom from tuberculosis only 30,000
are adult workmen—although 40,000 would
probably be nearer the mark—we obtain another nine million pounds lost every year to the
nation. ' This added to the other two items
makes up sixteen million pounds a year lost
by tuberculosis; and there are many other
sources of loss, in lameness, in recoveries after
long illness and inability in cases which do
not die, in tuberculous animals slaughtered,
in necessary inspection, and so on, which need
not here be enumerated and calculated out.

Another method of getting at the total loss
is that tuberculosis, as has been calculated by
actuaries, reduces the expectation of life of
every inhabitant of the country by two and a
half years, when the diminution of life duration
is distributed all round. Now, taking man,
woman, and child, the average income of the
wage-earning classes is about £23 a year per
individual, and in our total 44 to 45 millions
of population there are about 38 millions
consisting of wage-earners. Multiplying 38
millions by 23 and again by $2\frac{1}{2}$, we obtain
2185 million pounds as the wages earned; and
if we take about two-thirds of this as the sum
necessary to adequately support the 38 millions
for the two and a half years, we obtain at least
700 million pounds as the capital value to
the nation of total eradication of consumption,
which, at 3 per cent. interest, means an annual

saving of 21 million pounds. This eradication, as we shall see, can be *guaranteed* for an expenditure of less than ten million pounds a year, for ten years, further expenditure almost stopping at the end of that period.

A calculation by Dr. Hermann Bigg,[1] Medical Officer of Health of New York City, made in 1903, estimates the annual loss to that city due to tuberculosis at 23,000,000 dollars, or £4,600,000, a year. The estimated total annual number of deaths in the whole United States is 150,000 people, representing an annual financial loss, calculated on the same basis as for New York City, of 330,000,000 dollars, or £66,000,000. On the same basis, the 75,000 deaths from all forms of tuberculosis in the United Kingdom in 1908, the last year for which we have figures, would cost exactly half the bill of the United States, or £33,000,000.

Another enormous national bill which would be almost entirely wiped away by a National Health Army is that which might be grimly described as the bill for the slaughter of the innocents.

One person out of every five persons born dies before the fifth birthday is reached, and under proper conditions of sanitation and healthy living at least eighty per cent. of these deaths could be avoided. Latin names figure in the returns of the Registrar-General as the

[1] Quoted from Latham and Garland, " Conquest of Consumption " (Fisher Unwin, 1910), p. 121.

cause of death, but in plain English the children die from dirt, ignorance, carelessness, and starvation. Also, sad to relate, there has not been the slightest improvement in this respect within the past forty years. Neither is it possible to hug the fond delusion that these are weak, enfeebled children, to preserve whom would deteriorate and enfeeble the race. These children who die are born healthy, and placed in similar circumstances any other children would succumb just as fast as these. The diseases of infancy fall upon the fit and the unfit; and epidemic diarrhœa, or bronchitis caused by neglect after measles, kill the fit just as much as the unfit. Just as in the case of the adults, infection with tubercle bacilli kills the fittest as well as the feeblest. The healthy have not been seized by tuberculosis because they have not been sufficiently exposed to infection, and the infection of tuberculosis comes up from the slums and slum-life, where it is cultivated and propagated by our present system of neglect.

Filth and filth infection causes nine-tenths of the preventable deaths occurring before the age of sixty-five, and if we join in this crusade for a National Health Army to help the poor, we help ourselves at the same time.

Time was when that filth disease, smallpox, claimed in the palace as its victim a French king, and at another the consort of a British monarch; as it was then with smallpox so is

it now with phthisis, and it is our duty to
see that as it now is with smallpox so shall
it be within the next ten years with phthisis.

So much for the doctrine of survival of the
unfittest as a result of the stamping out of
disease in general, and infantile slaughter in
particular; let us now look at the economic
effect of allowing a state of affairs to persist
under which one life in five is destroyed before
five years of life have run.

In the first place, there is the cost of pro-
duction of these children, the drain on the
mother's strength and energy, the extra food,
the nursing, the doctors' bills, and all wasted in
sorrow and bitterness of heart. But of more
importance to the nation is the wrongful age
distribution caused by this infant slaughter as
between workers and non-workers of the community. This inordinate infantile death-rate,
about ten times as great as the rest of the
population, leaves us with a much dispropor-
tionate number of non-earning children to be
supported by the workers. Just at the period
hardest for family maintenance, on account of
this enormous death-rate, there are too many
small mouths to fill, and too few growing up to
earning ages to help the toil-worn father with
his task of keeping a home together.

A certain order of social economist talks of
the necessity of keeping up the birth-rate, but
as long as present social conditions persist this
is but adding fuel to a consuming fire.

We could have a happier, healthier, and wealthier people of equal population with little more than half the present birth-rate, if we looked after the death-rate with an efficient National Health Army.

Let us look after the death-rate and the birth-rate will take care of itself. There are even now nearly twice as many births as deaths in our country, and the wonder is where to find, at any rate under present social conditions, employment and maintenance for our ever-increasing population.

Improve social conditions by attending to health, and all this vicious circle of over-production and slaughtering of children will disappear automatically by the operation of a fundamental biological law ; the natural law will assert itself that as you improve the condition of the people they will reproduce less rapidly, but we shall get a more virile race, with a less proportion of children to adults. Birth-rate and death-rate will both go down together, which is the best economic and social result which could possibly exist.

Meanwhile the slaughter of the children goes on unchecked, and as a strange result, most paradoxical but most true, we have to maintain at least one-third more children between the age of infancy and five years than we ought to have ; these luckless infants have to be maintained by the productive work of the nation, and the cost estimated in money is certainly not less than £1,000,000 sterling every year.

At least 100,000 children lose their lives every year from preventable causes, which we do nothing to make impossible. Did we ask the fond mothers of some of these lost children their value, we might be told they were " worth their weight in gold "; but if, on the economic basis of what they have cost, and leaving out of account their future productive value to the nation, we set them down as equivalent to £10 each, we obtain the sum of £1,000,000 a year.

These two instances of tuberculosis and infantile mortality have been selected to show what disease costs in money every year; dozens of other diseases, less heavy in their incidence but mounting up in their totality, might be put forward along similar lines. The two that have been quoted, together cost us more than double the price of an effective national service for their prevention; and hence, provided it can be shown that prevention would be effectual, a clear case has been made out on the basis of economics alone for taking action in this matter.

CHAPTER II

THE FOLLIES OF OUR PRESENT PUBLIC HEALTH SERVICE

THE reader of the previous chapter has probably come to the conclusion that the object of the writer is to convert all, or the great majority of, medical men into medical officers of health on the system now in vogue on a smaller scale under our municipalities and county authorities. To this the reply of the writer is, " Heaven forbid ; " his object is the prevention of disease, and any system less likely to achieve this object than our present wretched Public Health System, or rather lack of all system, he cannot well imagine. Such a system of how-not-to-do-it far surpasses the Circumlocution Office in its wild and ludicrous absurdity.

No attack whatever is intended upon the personnel of the Medical Officers of Health of the Country, but a new National Medical Service must be formed, and the present heterogeneous collection of absurdity and impotence removed, if any true progress is to be made in safeguarding the National Health.

The difficulty is to know where to make a start in attacking this colossal Castle of

Humbug that we call our Public Health Service. Let us commence with a particular example.

Quite in recent times, a Corporation of over 300,000 citizens required what is called an M.O.H., that is to say, a Medical Officer of Health. They wanted, it will be noted, *one* medical officer of health to prevent disease ravaging these 300,000 people, a task which, if undertaken with any approach to seriousness, would require at least 150 to 200 medical men. But in this, strange to say, they were in nowise peculiar, for that is the custom all over the country, so let us pass over this ludicrous aspect as too common to excite our risible faculties. The next point is that the Corporation in question offered the magnificent salary of £600 for this Medical Officer; for, of course, he would have a good deal to do in preserving the health of 300,000 people. Now, in spite of the arduous duties, the Corporation might have had the services of men well trained in exactly the type of work required; they might have picked and chosen from amongst many men who had for years executed such duties in other large Corporations; but the Corporation, acting through its City Council, thought it might be better to have a local man with some knowledge perhaps of the individual constitutions peculiar to the 300,000 odd people who inhabited this city, so they chose a worthy gentleman who, in addition to being up till then a private general medical practitioner, had recently been a City Father, or, in other words, a City Councillor.

The City Councillors knew him well, and knew they could work harmoniously with him, and he with them; besides, his predecessor had likewise been chosen from the ranks of the City Fathers, with eminent success.

The result has clearly demonstrated the wisdom of the choice; the health of that city is excellent—it is by no means the highest in its death-rate amongst our great cities, and there has been no observable increase in death-rate during the few years that have elapsed since the appointment.

What is the moral?

The moral might be that no prolonged experience as Medical Officer of Health is necessary in appointing to such an important post, provided you can obtain a man who has acquired experience and tact by service on the City Council; but it might also be that the experience and ability of the Medical Officer of Health matter very little under present conditions as far as the Health of the City is concerned.

There is both humour and pathos in this plain true tale; the humour is that it did not matter, the pathos that it should not matter.

Yet the position of Medical Officer of Health of a large city is no sinecure; his duties are most multifarious, and although a great many are carried out by deputies, the situation requires great tact and a good deal of knowledge for successful treatment.

But, as a matter of fact, by far the greater part of the work requires little or no medical knowledge, and could be done as well by an astute solicitor's clerk as by a medical man.

As far as his official duties at present are concerned, the Medical Officer of Health simply is an administrator of an ill-assorted collection of Laws, some good and others bad and incomplete, supposed to be all that is necessary for the due maintenance of Public Health and prevention of disease. Meanwhile, if we may personify Disease, we can truly say that it laughs and jeers at us and our Public Health Acts and Medical Officers of Health and their Sanitary Inspectors, not merely in our slums, but in all our public places, and carries off to premature deaths every year at least 300,000 persons, whom an organised State Public Health Service could preserve as sound and healthy lives.

It is true that there are, here and there, Medical Officers of Health who exceed their Commission, because they are keen on their work and introduce reforms as far as they can get backing from their local authorities; but it is not in the Bill, and voluntary effort can do little or nothing towards tackling the larger problems of disease prevention.

The fundamental condition of reform is that the whole aspect and outlook of (1) Government, (2) Public, (3) Private Medical Practitioner, and (4) Public Health Officer must be radically and completely changed.

We do not require an extension and amplification of the present systems or any branches of them, but a new system, including in organic co-ordination the Private Practitioners; the Hospitals, Voluntary and Poor Law, and their Staffs; the Infectious Diseases and Municipal Hospitals and their Staffs; the Dispensaries, Public and Provident; the District Medical Officers and Relieving Officers; and the present so-called Public Health Service.

We require a Cosmos evolved out of this Chaos.

Order cannot be evolved out of chaos until this heterogeneous mass of machinery is set in gear, and driven by one motive-power managed by one overseeing intelligence.

Till this has been achieved, waste of money and human energy, and impotence to handle and prevent disease, must coexist side by side, as every sociologist who has studied the subject admits they do at the present moment.

The National Medical Service, to be at all co-ordinated and effective, must be truly National, and not merely a congeries of Municipal Services out of touch with one another. There must be provision at each local centre for the direction of local affairs, and every particle of useful voluntary service on City Councils and Hospitals can be, and ought to be, utilised as at present, or, rather, much more than at present ; but the medical men must be part of a service as truly National in its scope as any of our present great civil or military National Services.

A young medical officer entering this service should have the opportunity of seeing service in all parts of the country, and being called by a local authority from any one part to any other ; and after the Service has once been established there must be no irregular admissions. The National Medical Service should be made one of the finest in the country, for none in the country would be more fundamental or essential, and the honours and emoluments should be such as to attract the finest brain-power of the youth of the nation.

The main objects of the National Medical Service should be twofold—(1) To give nstruction in the laws of hygiene and healthy living, sowing this knowledge broadcast in both school and workshop ; and (2) to take effective steps to stamp out infectious diseases, armed with compulsory powers for this purpose.

Nearly all disease is due either to unhealthy habits of life, or to infection from other individuals pursuing unhealthy habits or living under unhealthy conditions. Wipe out these two fundamental causes, and the number of diseased individuals left to be " doctored " would shrink to such dimensions that our hospitals would be well-nigh empty, and our National

Chest correspondingly fuller of treasure for other good work.

Let us look for a moment at the question of how these two fundamental objects of a national health service are carried out now by all the disunited branches of the medical profession, both private and public.

By long odds, the more important of the two functions is the educative one, for if the mass of the people could be taught in a real practical way the elementary laws of healthy living and what made for good health and what for disease, there would be no delay in introducing reforms for prevention of infection.

The Government that refused to take adequate action, once the people saw what was required, would soon be swept out of existence, and replaced by one that would carry out reform.

Now, what attempts are at present being made to give the people this education; what is the medical profession doing in public health service or in private practice, and what is being done by educated laymen? The answer is simple: there is no concerted action whatever, nothing in the way of a national effort. A few posters on the walls of our slums about temperance, and feeding babies; notices not to spit in our public conveyances; occasional and sporadic attempts at "Health Lectures"; tuberculosis crusades with limelight views, and lectures. Very good, all of it, and much to be commended; but as an attempt at a national effort to educate the people in the laws of health—well, one can only repeat some of the responses to the Litany over it, in great sorrow of spirit.

Let us wake up and be truly ashamed of ourselves, and start to teach some practical hygiene in our schools as a compulsory and important subject. Let us teach our school teachers first some of the principles of how health is preserved, so that they know more about the little bodies they have to look after physically as well as mentally, and so do not treat them as disembodied minds. Let us start our newly appointed School Medical Officers as teachers as well as inspectors, and see if they can prevent some children falling ill, in addition to writing reports on those already afflicted. This is no sneer at work well begun, but rather to say let us do more of it.

Next let us take most of our 32,000 qualified medical practitioners and turn them loose on the slums as missionaries of health, as a change and relaxation from pottering in vain at disease so far advanced as to be beyond their skill.

It is a peculiar irony of fate that the very name of "doctor" means a teacher, and yet he never, or very rarely, teaches nowadays, but earns his living chiefly by pouring medicines into people who would in most cases be better without them.

The average poor person, as also many who are not poor save in intelligence, goes to the "doctor" for "medicine," and the doctor panders

to the prejudice and gives " medicine." He can
scarcely help himself; if he gave no " medicine "
he would soon have but little practice. Advice
thrown in gratis may be good, and after all you
need not take it if you do not want it; but
it is certainly the " medicine " that is going to
make you well, that is what costs the doctor
something, and that is what you pay your fee
for, and expect to have.

Yet the doctors themselves complain of
quackery and the undoubted frauds of patent-
medicine vending and advertising. Why, the
people are only bettering their instruction, for
the doctors, by their actions if not their words,
lay such stress on the " bottle " that it becomes
the essential thing to the patient's mind. He
sees a well-written piece of quackery in a news-
paper advertisement, a widely-cast net which
includes his symptoms, and he imagines the
others he has not got; this represents to him
the doctor's palaver. Is it any wonder that he
sends for the essential thing from his point of
view, to wit, the " medicine "? After all, will it
do him much more harm, or good, than the
rapidly thrown together " bottle " supplied at
the dispensary of the private practitioner who
sees forty patients in an hour at a shilling a
head? Truly, the medical profession has itself
to blame for many of the evils which have come
upon it.

The medical profession requires sadly to have
some dignity put back into it by being made a

truly teaching profession, as the popular name
of its exponents indicates.

Many medicines are most valuable, and need
not be taken in homœopathic doses when their
use is really indicated. There is only one
greater medical fraud than homœopathy, and
that is faith-healing. But, at the same time, if
doctors could see their way to give one-tenth
the present amount of drugging and ten times
the amount of teaching, it would be better both
for the world at large and the self-respect of the
medical profession.

Turning to the second fundamental purpose
of a National Medical Service, viz. the prevention of infection, how do we find that provided
for at the present time? Here we do find legislation existent which attempts to place the
Medical Officer of Health in some co-ordination with the Medical Practitioner. The best
possible attempt, it may be, which can be made
under present conditions; but the most elementary examination of its mode of operation and
restraining effect upon the spread of disease is
sufficient to convince any one with an open
mind that it is but a miserable *pis aller*, that
would not be tolerated for a moment did we
possess a real National Medical Service armed
with powers to proceed on the offensive against
infectious diseases.

The present mechanism is that any medical
practitioner who has seen a case which he has
diagnosed as an attack of one of certain types

of infectious diseases is compelled to notify
the same to the Public Health Authority;
and unless he can certify that the case can be
properly isolated and attended at home, the
Public Health Authority has power to remove
it to a Public Infectious Diseases Hospital.
Usually in the case of poor people the case is
so removed, if there is room, at the time being,
in the Hospital.

To the lay mind this may sound perfectly
all right, but there is little doubt that it costs
lives by the ten thousand annually, and is one
of the most puerile ways of dealing with a
most serious problem which can well be imagined. Especially in the case of children's
diseases does this hold good, and it is a conservative estimate to say that in infectious
diseases peculiar to childhood this nefarious
system costs the country fifty thousand lives
annually.

Observe, in the first place, that here, where
the safety of the community is at stake and
the spread of infection is to be prevented, the
machinery is first set in action by some ignorant
lay person, living in all probability in a dirty
slum, and entirely uneducated in matters of
health and disease.

Neither the medical practitioner nor the
public health officer has any commission to
go forth and find the disease, not even when
an epidemic is on; no—the disease must come
to the doctor. The enemy must walk past

our outposts and into our camp, and ask to be attacked and arrested, before we stir hand or foot. Is not the whole thing too ludicrous for the serious consideration of any one but the witch-doctor or medicine-man of a savage tribe? It is reminiscent of the days of burning for witchcraft or healing by incantations and charms.

If we really believe in this as a modern method of combating infectious disease, let us at least show some charity to those just a shade less advanced in intelligence than ourselves, who cultivate the pious art of faith-healing and swallow the miracles of Lourdes.

The patient reports to the doctor, and the doctor reports to the medical officer of health, and the medical officer of health reports to the infectious diseases hospital,[1] and then, if there is room, the ambulance is sent for the patient. Meanwhile, the disease germs have not been reporting at all, but have been going on with their business, and next day there is another case to be removed from the same house or the house next door, after "the tale of the house that Jack built" has been run through again. Is it any wonder that we have epidemics of acute infectious diseases?

It is to be remembered that nine-tenths of the disease is situated in the low-class, closely crowded property of slum-land, where

---

[1] "And the parson told the sexton, and the sexton tolled the bell."

the people are poor, ignorant, and perhaps
sometimes careless of what to do, and that bad
cases have often run a good deal of their infectious course, and had contact with a good
many susceptible persons, before ever a doctor
has seen them at all. The poor hard-working
wife of the labourer, with all her family and
housework to attend to, may be forgiven if
she fails to understand even for two or three
days that what she thinks is a cold or sore
throat in one of her children is the beginning
of a serious infectious disease, and there is no
one going round inquiring for sick children
in the houses, even when it is known that a
severe epidemic is in progress. No; the free-
born Briton must be allowed to infect his
neighbours in peace, and undisturbed by any
domiciliary visits of a Health Authority. He
is not permitted to neglect the mind of his
child, but he can practically neglect the body,
and its care and requirements, to his heart's
content.

The infectious ailments of the middle and
upper classes practically all originate in this
way in the lower classes, and are carried up
by casual contacts in a hundred ways: by
contacts made on the street; in public buildings, in public conveyances; through food and
clothing which has been in contact in the slums,
and so on. In nothing so much as in infectious
disease is it really true that we *are* our brother's
keeper, and that "no man liveth to himself,

and no man dieth to himself"; there is but
one set in all Nature of infective organisms,
which produce the same results in the bodies
of rich and poor alike, and we cannot be
healthy as long as our poor brother in the slum
is afflicted. Both common humanity and self-
interest call out loudly to us to help him, and
we have just seen how we have been doing it.

The better-circumstanced classes suffer less
severely from infectious disease, not because
they are immune, but because they are brought
less in contact with it, in the first place; and,
secondly, because they are better nursed and
cared for when it falls upon them. For example, fatality from measles is very rare in
middle or better class practice, but it is one of
the most dangerous and fatal of diseases in
slum-land, because of the want of care. By
far the greater number of cases are never seen
by a doctor at all; the children are allowed to
infect any other susceptible children about them
in a wholesale fashion; there is scarcely any
attempt at isolation, proper feeding, nursing, or
after-attention, and a doctor is only called in
when the child is choking in bronchitis, or past
help almost from some other sequel arising from
the want of care.

Is it any wonder, then, that 20,000 children
die every year of measles alone; nearly as many
more of whooping cough, and twice as many
of epidemic diarrhœa? Until we have our
properly organised National Medical Service,

C

this hideous sacrifice of at least 90,000 children every year is going on, and bound to continue. When we get our service it can be stopped.

In the second place, the present Public Health Service is defective and incomplete in that certain infectious diseases, and these often most dangerous, are not even compulsorily notifiable at all. For example, infantile or epidemic diarrhœa, the most dangerous disease of infants in the summer months, and with a frightfully high mortality, is not notifiable, and most of the poor little sufferers only reach hospital when they are utterly collapsed and there is absolutely no chance of saving them.

More remarkable still, that disease which in our country slays double the number of any other, viz. tuberculosis, has until recently not been a notifiable disease. Even now it is permissible to the Local Authority to say whether it is to be notifiable or not; and even when it is made notifiable the whole object of notification is stultified by the fact that *no action follows on notification*. The Local Health Authority has no power to isolate without the full consent of the patient, who has *carte blanche* to go on infecting new sacrifices for the microbe of this dread disease all around him. Nor would it be of much value for any one Local Authority to attempt to deal properly with tuberculosis, if it was being infected by invasion from the areas of other Local Authorities all round, producing an effect like the thistle-down from the lazy man's farm alongside falling upon the ground of the thrifty. This question is one for the Nation, not for local authorities, either Poor Law or Municipal or County.

But tuberculosis, with its annual national tribute of seventy-five thousand lives, and the way it can be conquered, is worthy of a chapter to itself, so we shall only point it out here as one amongst the many diseases against which no *effectual* steps are at present being taken by our present Public Health Service.

From all that has been said, it will be seen that we possess no Public Health Service worthy of the name, even we Anglo-Saxons who possess the reputation of leading the World in matters of Hygiene.

As well might we send forth the privateers and letters-of-marque of Queen Elizabeth's time to fight the modern navy of our most powerful rival, as go on with our present equipment for offensive action against disease, and hope or pray for a victory.

All honour to the wooden walls of England and to the memory of the brave men who fought within them, but their day is over; and all honour to our Municipalities and medical officers of health, and the private donors who have supported our Voluntary Hospitals like the old privateers, and fought the good fight against disease in the face of long odds. But the day of these things is passing away. Science has shown us a better and more excellent way; our pioneers have found out how to win the long-contested battle if we only possess the grit to organise and send forward a disciplined army.

Let us once more lead forward the whole world on the glorious path to health and happiness as we have done of yore.

CHAPTER III

THE DOCTOR AND HIS PATIENT IN PRIVATE PRACTICE AND IN STATE PRACTICE

So far we have been concerned with medical science in relationship to the health and welfare of the community as a whole; a subject which intimately concerns each separate individual, because, as we have seen, the health of each person is dependent upon the health of others from whom his infection with disease arises.

It is a remarkable fact, in view of all we know as to causation of disease, that we have allowed matters so to drift on in our civilised communities that the first line of attack and defence is manned by less than ten per cent. of the medical profession, while over ninety per cent. are intermittently engaged as work turns up, upon what might be described as a guerilla warfare with disease after the enemy has thoroughly invaded and occupied the country.

Under anything approaching a normal and scientific condition of affairs these proportions ought to be exactly reversed, and eighty to ninety per cent. of medical men should be organised in a great service carrying out measures on the offensive against disease, while the smaller proportion of ten to twenty per cent. might still be engaged in carrying out such work as arose from disease which had escaped the attention of the regular State service. Or the smaller proportion might bear the same relationship to the State service as the secondary school teacher does to the primary school teacher—that is to say, attend more especially to those who, better supplied with means, desired a separate and more exacting service from the main bulk of the population.

There is little question that a national service must arise in the end out of the general sickness and invalidity scheme now being contemplated by the Government. For when once conditions of medical service for the great bulk of the people have been simplified and placed on a common basis all over the country, and the payment for this medical service is made by Government out of a fund in part contributed by the workmen and in part by taxation, it will be obvious to the powerful and unified organisation working such a scheme that both the more economical and the more scientific way of dealing with disease is to catch it early and stop it at its source.

The scheme will, however, end in disastrous failure if it is allowed to drift as to its management into the hands of dozens of so-called Friendly Societies, all acting on different principles, and in competition with one another, instead of being kept in the hands of the Government.

The scheme is at present only intended to include workmen, but later it will inevitably be extended to wives and families, after which we may expect the National Medical Service to develop rapidly by a quite obvious process of evolution in which different branches of service become specialised amongst the staff of the now universal system of State Medical Insurance.

At the present time, however, we have to deal with the fact that over eighty per cent. of the medical profession are engaged in practice for fees or payments made by the patient, and in this chapter the object is to examine whether or not this arrangement is advantageous to individual and community; whether it is an economical system in money and in health; and, most important of all, how it is affected by modern social and economic conditions of labour. We shall see that for the bulk of the people its death-knell is already being rung, and that it is becoming so inefficient under the action of small local co-operative systems, clubs, societies, and tontines, that it is making the name of medical science a disgrace. It is turning doctors' private practices into fraudulently conducted business concerns in which the doctor loses all dignity and self-respect, and the patient is cheated of that advice and treatment which he imagines is being given to him, and upon which his very life may depend.

Just as there is no service more valuable, and honourable, and worthy of high reward than that conscientiously rendered by a skilful doctor to his patient, so, and to the same degree, there is no greater dis-service, in fact, no greater crime, than scamped and inefficient medical attention, than want of care in diagnosis and proper treatment, or negligence in possessing that knowledge which the progress of medicine demands.

Consider for a moment how helpless the patient is in the hands of the doctor, how little he is able to form any just estimate of his doctor's skill and knowledge of the matter in hand, how wholly reliant in pure faith upon his doctor, the patient must be. Strong as the Roman Catholic's belief in the infallibility of Mother Church, as represented in the father-confessor, must be the patient's reliance on Medical Science as represented by his physician. Knowledge of right or wrong in medicine the patient has none ; his only refuge is faith in his doctor.

Seeing that this is so, how high ought the ideal of medical practice to be, and how great is the personal responsibility of the doctor to each patient he examines. His duty demands that his examination and care of the case shall be all that his ability and knowledge can make it. There must be no scamping of work, no hurrying, no superficiality.

Now, there is, unfortunately, little question

that in a very large share of private practice in this country, and much more so in many hospitals, these conditions do not obtain, work is habitually scamped, and patients defrauded of that which they are in many cases doing their poor best to pay for, and imagine that they are getting.

This holds particularly amongst practice in the working-class districts where fees are small, and the share of medical work so performed is increasing rapidly year by year, as dispensary practices go on multiplying, as clubs, tontines, and friendly societies go on flourishing and growing, and as in one way or another doctors are cheated and scamped in their fees all over the country, and forced to work under conditions in which good workmanship is well-nigh impossible.

This statement does not apply to all working-class practices; there are hundreds of doctors working amongst the poor who charge fair and reasonable fees for their work, and carry out their work conscientiously and well; but there are also hundreds of the other type who accept fees for which good work is utterly impossible. It is this latter class who are a disgrace to the profession, and are not merely reducing it to a purely mercenary business, but are fraudulently imposing upon the poor dupes who are their patients, by taking money under false pretences.

The working classes lend themselves to this chicanery by trying to obtain cheap medical attention by going to the sixpenny or shilling doctor, or by trying to screw the doctor by means of their club or sick benefit society. The doctor agrees to see them for a miserable pittance, and he does see them, gives them a bottle, and nothing more. It is a very cheap system and a very nasty one.

The last thing in this world to have cheap is medical advice, and the sooner the public gets to know it the better. If the layman will be a fool, let him go to a cheap tailor, or even to a cheap lawyer; he may live to learn to know better; but never to a cheap doctor, or he may never discover his mistake.

But, it may be said, the workman cannot afford the fees charged by a good doctor; let us be patient and go on with the chapter; we may find some solution for his case also—although it is not in the voluntary club; that club is only fit to kill him, not cure him.

This system of cheap, low-class medical work in so-called dispensary practice, or by contract work for clubs, etc., is not only incapacitating and killing thousands of working people every year, it is thoroughly ruining, in character, moral fibre, and income, the medical profession itself. It is a debasing and malignant process, sinking deeper and spreading wider all the time, and although by working themselves to death, or by employing raw or ignorant hack assistants, a few men make big incomes, a much larger number of men are merely existing in great poverty, and always on the verge of financial disaster.

This is well known within the profession, where the contract system is almost universally detested on account of its many vices for both practitioner and public; but the public has not begun to realise it, and the system, on account of its cheapness, has caught on in the thickly populated manufacturing districts and towns.

The medical man is caught in this whirlpool, and cannot help himself. In very many districts the choice is between taking contract work— indeed, begging and toadying for it—or not doing enough practice to keep the wolf from the door.

A large number of medical men are only able to curse and rail at this contract practice, and mistakenly think that the proposed Governmental system of sickness and invalidity insurance would only be an extension of it. It would be worth their while to consider how it has come to pass that all these benefit societies of all types, and clubs of all species, have come into existence, and try to see what it all means, and what is the way out. Continued vituperation of a system that not only members of the medical profession, but all educated men and sociologists who have examined it, admit to be bad, serves no useful purpose. It is already sufficiently damned; let us examine how it comes to be there, what it means, and what is the salvation. Let us do this not only in our own interests, but in those of the unfortunate patients who, in a different way, are suffering as much as the medical profession.

The origin of these various forms of local amalgamation into medical benefit societies of all types, is the same as that which centuries ago formed our national clans and noble families; which founded the Nations of Students in our mediæval Universities; which united our apprentices into Guilds, and gave origin to our City Companies; which gave the power to feudal chiefs, and gathered communities into free boroughs. In our own day, the same guiding spirit has led to combinations as diverse from each other in purpose as our Trades Unions on the one hand, and our gigantic commercial Trusts on the other.

The principle, in fact, lies at the root of the whole of our civilisation, and is as deep-seated as the principle of organic evolution itself. Men have discovered that combination and unity give strength and power to carry out projects utterly impossible to the individual.

Such combinations are seldom wholly good or wholly evil in their consequences, and whether on the whole they are good or evil depends upon their reaction upon the community or communities either employing them or affected by their influence.

Some of the evils of contract medical practice to both contracting parties have been pointed out above, but there are certain compensating advantages which might be caused to increase enormously under a better and wider system, and all or nearly all of the disadvantages might be made to disappear.

In the first place, it may be pointed out that for the greater part of the wage-earning class, including all the unskilled and a great share of the partially skilled labour of the country, the only alternative to the Sick Club is the workhouse and Poor Law treatment or the Out-patient Department of a Charity Hospital, and, as we shall see in a later chapter, this is worse than the club system.

The numbers of the population involved in this category run into several millions—probably thirty-eight millions would be a conservative estimate—out of our total forty-five millions.

While the head of a family can himself keep at work he may possibly be able to pay low fees to a doctor for attendance on his wife or child; but when he himself is seriously ill and has to give up work for any length of time, only for his trade-union sick pay and sick-club medical attendance he would soon be destitute.

Think how many families are struggling along with the father earning eighteen shillings a week, and occasionally out of work, and only small children still at school; how many more have to subsist on less than thirty shillings a week all told; and how are these to make better provision against misfortune in the shape of that ill-health to which they, from their environment, are more exposed than any other class in the nation, than by the few pence subscribed weekly to the sick-club? They cannot possibly do more, and those better circumstanced who inveigh against the thriftlessness and extravagance of the poor should first of all try to put themselves in their position. If there be added some consideration of their education and development, some thought of how little chance they have ever had of seeing what thrift and pinching can ultimately produce in the way of better conditions and increased comfort, we might be able to pardon some of their shortcomings. Let us think of the sordid surroundings, the hard struggle to keep above water, the comfortlessness of it all, and the endlessness of it, and we may forgive them breaking down on pay-day and snatching an illusory happiness which a day later but sinks them deeper down.

The writer is no sentimentalist, no believer in charity; he earnestly desires the worker to participate in his own upraising. If we cannot develop moral fibre and courage in these people we cannot help them. But let us set about it aright; do not let us ask them to undertake impossibilities under a system which is dragging them down and submerging them. If the point of view be altered so as to obtain a better perspective, it may perhaps be seen that these vices of the poorest are part and parcel of their condition, just as certainly as the symptoms and mental attitude of the diseased man are part of his disease.   Get the system of living improved, and the individual will improve with it; he may never be an angel, but he may be less of a devil if he be less tormented.

Biology teaches us that there are two fundamental things in all life, the organism and its past and present environment; the two react on each other, and probably the environment has more power in changing the organism than the organism has in altering the environment, but both can and do react.   Now, in regard to the man in the slum, we men higher up out of the slum have been expecting the slum man (*i.e.* the organism) to do all the altering, and have not been paying enough attention to altering the environment.   We have had all our eyes on the human being, preaching to him of better things and trying to alter him, and when we have failed we have usually cursed him as a thing too vile to live, and left it at that. When we have touched the environment at all, we have done it usually by charity in all its many useless forms, and of these the present Poor Law is the worst.   It is just about time we set about considering in a really philosophical way, as a scientific people attacking a scientific problem, how to improve the creature's environment and give him a better system of things to work in.   Not an exotic system, be it remarked, but a natural workaday one, which, once started, will go on improving itself.   We can do this better if we put all our fine feelings and sentimentality and charity in our pockets, and find out what is wrong.

As an example of this very principle in one of its not least important aspects, we may take the club system of medical practice of which we have been talking, and study how to improve it. Disease and its aftermath lead to more destitution, submerging of the poor, and filling of the workhouse and its accessories than anything else, so that the problem is worth tackling.

If, as we have seen, joining a sick benefit club is the only insurance against ill-health that the workman can provide himself with during health, we may take it that he does not join simply to spite and defraud the doctor; it is simply a reaction to a particular environment.

The evils of the club system arise very simply. In the first place, the workmen are not able to pay enough to raise a sufficient sum to adequately repay the doctor for attending to so many. In the second place, the aggregate amount coming in annually as a fixed sum is nevertheless sufficient to tempt the doctor to undertake the club work, although in many cases he knows within his soul he is going to scamp it, both in time and attention, as compared with his better paid private work. Thirdly, the workers belonging to the club have eliminated all competition amongst themselves for the doctor's services, and have got better terms from the doctor, as far as money goes, in that he attends them much cheaper per visit than if each of them had gone to him separately when ill. At the same time, by their union and by the annual sum they have to offer, they have turned the tables and set the doctors of the district in competition, and by going about amongst the doctors and exciting this competition they have succeeded in getting their work done at the lowest possible figure per head per annum, and fondly imagine they have done a good stroke of business for themselves.

The end result is that the club sweats the doctor to the last drop, and the doctor in turn scamps the club patient's case to the last inch he can go, without losing his appointment, and in this process, as pointed out earlier in the chapter, the doctor is master of the situation, for he possesses knowledge, and ignorance possesses the patients.

By the operation of these simple processes, and a natural reaction of cause and effect, that vicious circle is established which renders club practice the detestation even of those doctors who engage in it, and at the same time such an unknown, but none the less terrible, evil to the poor sufferers who pay, albeit as little as they can help, for the ministrations of the physician.

What is the way out from all this chaos? Precisely that unified system of State insurance against sickness which so many members of the medical profession are at present deriding as an extension of club and contract practice.

D

An extension in one sense it certainly is, but not in that nefarious sense which the profession attaches to the word " contract " practice to-day.

In the first place, it is proposed that not only the workman, but also the employer and the State shall contribute ; so that there must be a larger sum to pay the doctor for adequate treatment and attendance. In the second place, the united income of the scheme is to be disbursed by the Government ; so that the State medical officer becomes a State servant, dealt with directly by the State and paid by the State, which is quite different to being paid by a motley crowd of Clubs and Friendly Societies. In the next place, the Government, being in charge of the scheme, can be approached by members of the State medical service for the institution of proper and equitable conditions of service. This cannot be done at all to the tens of thousands of Friendly Societies, which have for their object in life setting the doctors in competition to secure, almost regardless of quality, the lowest price possible. A Government could not afford to behave in this way ; the workmen, having once paid their subscriptions, would make it obvious that they must have a properly equipped and efficient service. A sweated service could not be this, and must inevitably tone up to the level of other national services.

It is a great mistake to compare a national medical insurance worked by Government with present conditions under the Poor Law, a system which stands condemned on many counts by all competent critics. Those defects in Poor Law administration which have caused other evils have also led to the degraded sweating of medical men by Poor Law Guardians. This system is seen at its acme of shoddiness in Ireland, in the vile treatment to which medical men have there been subjected time after time by ignorant Irish Poor Law Guardians.

There is no question that Boards of Poor Law Guardians are doomed, so that at the very least the officers of any public system of sickness insurance would be under more responsible bodies, administering larger areas in Boroughs and Counties. For this reason the control would be in the hands, at the very worst, of more enlightened people than at present.

It is just here, however, that the new medical service may lose much of its efficiency if it is not made a truly national one. If the new medical service is placed under municipal control it will lose its coherence, and become like a territorial army of many isolated units, instead of one unified National Army of Health.

The Scylla and Charybdis to be avoided in the projected reform are the Friendly Societies, which are very anxious to either wreck, or themselves administer the scheme, on the one hand, and the Municipalities and other Local Authorities on the other.

The true solution is one National Service for

the whole country, under a Minister of Public Health of Cabinet rank. Local conditions for hospitals and administration may be left in the hands of local authorities, but the medical officers must be appointed to a National Service and be transferable from one local centre to another, and open to promotion from one place to another.

Nor would the annual sum required be at all enormous to thoroughly carry out such a national scheme of State Insurance against disease.

There are just over 32,000 medical men in practice in the United Kingdom of Great Britain and Ireland. It is quite a liberal estimate to take the average income of the profession at £250 per annum; it has been quoted at £200 per annum. On the basis of £250 each per annum, the aggregate income of the whole of the medical profession accordingly amounts to just eight million pounds. The profession is at present underpaid, when the professional training and its duration and expense are taken into account, so that if we add one-fourth more for this, so as to make the State National Medical Service attractive for good men, we arrive at the net result that the State can employ all of these 32,000 medical men at a total cost of ten millions per annum. The average annual pay for each doctor would be somewhat over £300 a year, and taking it that a junior entered at about one hundred and fifty pounds a year, this would mean a system rising on ordinary promotions and good service to a maximum of one thousand pounds, and a small number of administrative officers at higher salaries, in the most distinguished posts.   It would form a magnificent service, second to none other in the country.

Also, there would be more doctors than at present to cope with working-class work.   For we have supposed *all* the men now in practice to enter the new service on full-time work. But not more than two-thirds of those now in private practice are engaged on working-class practice.   Accordingly, the national cost could either be reduced one-third in amount to six and two-third millions annually, one-third of the profession electing to remain on in private work ; or, alternatively, a much more effective service could be instituted at the above cost of ten millions annually.   Now, when it is remembered that (1) workmen contribute, (2) employers contribute, and (3) the State contributes, this amount is certainly not an excessive sum to raise for such an enormous boon as a complete full-time National Medical Service would mean to the Nation.

Let us look for a moment more closely at what the necessary contributions would mean to raise this sum.   There would, it is estimated, be 12,000,000 workmen participating in any scheme of compulsory State Insurance.   Suppose that each of these workmen contributed only one penny a week of insurance money, and the

employer contributed also one penny a week
for each workman he employed—surely not an
excessively grinding tax upon either. Then
the combined sum raised from these two sources
would be five million two hundred thousand
pounds annually, and the State would only have
to add one million four hundred thousand to
obtain the full and free services of the present
staff of doctors working for the poor, and for
a sum of four million eight hundred thousand could provide adequately and well for a
National Medical Service sufficient to attend
not merely to the workmen, but to every man,
woman, and child in the whole Kingdom, and
much better than is done at present.

The whole scheme is not nearly as costly as
the provision required under the Old Age Pen-
sions Act, which, long talked of, is now an
established fact; and there is no doubt that
the National Medical Service would prove at
least as beneficial and as popular as the Old
Folks' Charter.

An important fact, well worth remembering,
is that this taxation would not really be new
national expenditure, but rather a great saving
of money to the people. For the doctors have
even now to be paid by hook or by crook in
some fashion or other; and so, although the
workman had to contribute his penny a week,
he would then no longer have to pay the doctor,
and so would save money and provide against
the evil day of illness. The gain, in disease

stopped at incipient stages and in increased health and corresponding power of his work-people, together with regularity of work less interrupted by illness, would more than repay the employer for his contribution ; and, lastly, the immunity from infection and premature death, given by the operations of such a National Health Service, would most certainly repay many times over the general taxpayer for his moiety of the fund. Leaving the question of money, let us now glance at the economy of such a system from the scientific and sociological point of view.

If the Government provides a sickness in-surance scheme such as outlined above, prac-tically all the doctors will be paid sufficiently for full-time service for the Government, and so the system comes under a unified control. As a result, the members of the Staff can be located and assigned work according to the views of the Minister in charge of the ser-vice and his advisers. Accordingly, in the in-tervals of attending to cases of serious illness, accidents, etc., attention can be given to inspec-tion and instruction as outlined in previous chapters. The work can also be adequately divided up so that one man is not nearly idle while another is working himself to death over scamped, ill-done work ; and also the whole question of hospital abuse falls away, because the doctor working inside the hospital is a fellow and colleague of the doctor at work out in the slums sending in the serious cases to him, and is no longer robbing the doctor outside in practice of his livelihood.

Contrast this with the present disjointed order of things, where the doctor sits idle half his time behind his red lamp and brass door-plate waiting for the patient, and the patient in the slum, ill himself and infecting others, waits and dies in the absence of the doctor whom our wretched system will not allow to come to him.

Take the case of the young graduate in medicine who sets up his plate and lamp at a street corner, and waits for patients to drop in upon him. For a period varying from six months to a year, if he sets up as a shilling dispensary doctor, to one to three years in an ordinary intermediate type of general practice, or, still more, of five to ten years if he is attempting to become a consulting physician or surgeon—for all this period he does hardly anything, and for a still longer period his time is only very partially employed. Even the fairly busy practitioner later on, or the dispensary practice man who runs through cases at breakneck speed in the so-called surgery in the evening and does his round of visits in the morning, has plenty of time between whiles in which he could do other things, such as hospital work, or organised slum inspection for disease requiring removal or treatment; but our wretched, hide-bound system of private

practice, with its strange, nonsensical code of
ethics and professional etiquette, requiring a
modern Cervantes to set the world a-laughing
at it—this monstrous system permits no latitude
to the doctor; he must lie in waiting at his
own home for disease to come to him. Even
when it does come to him, it must come in
proper guise, and all formalities must be properly arranged before he can touch it.

A good part of the doctor's time is even
spent in secretarial work—in sending out and
collecting his bills for work done, and in getting
his collectors to look after bad debts for him.
An exception, of course, is the ready-money,
ready-made, shilling-dispensary-practice degradation, where the patient tips the doctor after
each little attention, and carries his bottle of
ill-assorted, harmless, useless physic back home
with him to drink in peace while he continues
uninterruptedly those evil courses which harbour
and encourage his disease.

How much preferable for the doctor to get
his quarterly cheque from Government, and
spend his time in being a doctor and looking
after questions of health and disease, leaving
bill-posting and fee-squeezing to those whose
business it is !

Again, under our present system the doctor
has absolutely no opportunity to keep himself
in touch with the progress of medical science,
and is apt to become a pure empiric, a quack
and a charlatan, who talks about, and pre-

tends a knowledge of, things of which he is profoundly ignorant. The doctor in general practice may be able to read occasionally in his weekly medical journal, or once upon a time attend a meeting of a local medical society; but this cannot adequately replace practical work in laboratory or hospital. From this latter source of stimulus and inspiration nine-tenths of our medical men are cut off from the day they qualify and cease to be medical students, till the day of their death in harness, struggling for their living and that of those dependent upon them.

The result is most deplorable, and greater than the lay public can possibly realise, or they would rise up in indignation and sweep the present system away wholesale, lock, stock, and barrel.

During the last fifteen to twenty years our knowledge on both medical and surgical sides has been increasing enormously, and for the same period the great majority of practitioners have been acquiring any acquaintance with new knowledge in a second or third hand way, and without any practical teaching.

Our present system provides no means by which, without losing their incomes, they can return for six months or a year to laboratory and hospital and have their minds refreshed by a post-graduate course. Many of them are so chronically steeped in ignorance that they do not even know that they require such a rejuvenation.

Nor are they to be blamed in the least; they are rather only to be pitied, and still more to be pitied are their patients, for whom it may be frankly admitted that they are conscientiously striving to do their best.

Contrast this state of affairs with what happens in the case of the medical officers of our Army and Navy and Indian Medical Services. Here there are modern, up-to-date Staff Colleges and Hospitals, to which the medical officers, after intervals of service, are allowed leave *on full pay*, to go and learn modern methods of diagnosis and treatment.

But the unfortunate general medical practitioner in private practice enjoys no such luxury as this; if he takes a short postgraduate course of two or three weeks, he must snatch it in a vacation, which he sadly needs for bodily recuperation, and no one offers to pay *his* fees, or work *his* practice and give him the money while he is taking the course.

Sad to have to state, in too many cases the private practitioner has almost ceased to be a professional man at all. He has become purely a business man, in a line of business which rarely yields more than a pittance.

There are, of course, very many who have not allowed the iron to enter into their souls, and in spite of the claims of a general practice, keep up an acquaintance with scientific medicine and modern practice. But the system is a horribly fossilising one, and the men who go asleep under it are scarcely to be blamed.

Another crying evil of our present system is the multitude of extraneous things, not related to professional skill in the remotest degree, which are necessary and make for success in the profession. It is often well known to his brother practitioners that the highly successful doctor, who has the largest and best-paying practice in the town or district, is by no means the best physician or surgeon in it. In fact, he is often little better than a well-qualified quack, who knows how to play on the feelings and sentiments of the laymen upon whose bodies he practises, because of the subtle influence he possesses over their minds.

The man who succeeds in general private practice is he who can best please the ladies, and who, by an affable exterior and calm pose of face, can hide the profound ignorance within his cranium, while his neighbour with tenfold the ability, but an abstracted or brusque manner, and without the social arts of pleasing, gets little or nothing to do.

Who are the jury to decide whether the doctor's work is done well or ill, but lay people who know nothing and can be taught nothing of the case? As to judgment by results, apart from egregious mistakes amounting to malpractice, how can the public judge here or determine how much is due to chance and how much to the ministrations of the doctor? If the case goes ill, an apt manner, carefully constructed statements, and sympathetic bearing convey the certainty that "the best possible has been done, but nature must have its course"; while if it goes well, "Oh, what skill! how well everything was done, and what a marvellous cure the doctor made of a bad case!"

In medical practice, so much necessarily rests on causes beyond control, that all depends on the impression upon lay minds produced by the doctor's manner as to the verdict upon him. This mental influence of the doctor on patient and patient's friends is sometimes valuable, when it is not used as a cloak for ignorance, but its absence is disastrous to the career of many a man who is lacking in the small social amenities, and in what might be called professional style, and yet possesses in high degree that professional skill and acumen which is essential in the treatment of serious disease. Also, it is most unfortunate when a plausible style covers, as it often does, lack of scientific ability, and the man depending upon his powers cultivates this manner as his chief stock-in-trade, instead of keeping himself up to date in his professional skill, and so becomes a mere charlatan, living upon the fact that most of the fees, especially in middle-class practice, are made from trivial, commonplace ailments, and calling in the consultant, or sending the case, if it is a poor patient, to hospital, as soon as he gets into any difficulties for which a competent practitioner would scorn asking assistance.

The final indictment against this system of private medical practice, even from the point of view of treatment and of the private patient, is the same as that which we have urged from the community's point of view in the prevention of disease, namely, that the most incompetent agent in the world for the purpose, to wit, the patient himself, sets the machinery in motion.

The patient is forced to go to the doctor either because he is enduring pain or because life, on account of weakness or depression, has become a burden to him.

Now, for both men and women, there are hundreds of cases where these indications only come in when it is too late to go to any doctor, and the case is beyond hope. This, too, where an earlier indication and visit to a competent doctor would have put quite a different complexion on the case.

Many most serious diseases, such, for example, as both phthisis and cancer, are frequently unattended by pain in their earlier stages, or even until far advanced, and it is far too late to go to the doctor when weakness and prostration have begun to supervene.

From our childhood we have been brought up, most of us, to associate a visit or inspection by the doctor with most unpleasant memories; partially due to the obnoxious habit of some physicians of pouring vile-tasting medicines into children, when there is no indication for them, and they are probably doing more harm than good, and, in great part also, from the fact that we scarcely ever see a doctor professionally unless there is something the matter either with ourselves or some one dear to us.

Why so often is it left to the doctor to pronounce a death sentence? Why is the doctor looked upon as a person only to be called in to exorcise disease? Would it not be a change for the better if we could get to look upon him as the Minister of Health rather than of Disease, and evolved a corresponding system?

It is in this saner way that educated people have within the last generation grown to regard another professional man who has made a special study of one branch of surgery, viz. the dentist. We no longer wait until we have violent toothache, and then rush off to the dentist to have the tooth extracted, as did our more immediate forefathers. We are learning that it is our duty to our children to take them once a year at least to the dentist to have their teeth inspected.

It would be a better day for most of us, even in regard to individual health as apart from public, if we learnt that our doctors ought to be preventive officers, and if we paid them an annual fee and went to be examined, and if necessary forewarned and treated, at periodical intervals.

How many men have learnt for the first

time that they were in the incipient or even more advanced stages of serious illness when they have gone to the doctor, as they imagined, in perfect health to be examined for life insurance; and how many, taking advantage of good advice given on such an occasion, have curbed a bad habit of life, or of appetite, and stopped an inroad of disease, which they would have only found out too late if they had gone to a doctor in the ordinary course of events?

No; the serious, unmistakable signs of disease, as visible or obvious to a laymen, often—too often—come too late to make that system, which leaves the individual sole arbiter of his health, a safe one, either for the patient himself, or for those immediately around him or dependent upon him, or for the general public.

We have seen how the unattended, often undiscovered, disease of slum-land reacts back upon the general health of the community. The same thing which holds for the community holds in still higher degree for the family; and that in all ranks, but more particularly in the lower classes, where families are huddled together and overcrowded.

How often do we see one sister after another in the same family dying of phthisis, or husband following wife, or wife husband, till a family is well-nigh wiped out? This, too, occurs where all possible care to avoid infection is taken by the family after the first member has gone to the doctor and had the case diagnosed. What is the cause of this, the most melancholy picture in all medical practice?

Nothing so much as the system which has for its fundamental basis that we do not go to our doctors until we think we are ill. The seeds of the fatal disease are often laid in the second and third members of the family before ᵔhe first has been to the doctor at all.

Think of it: only one person in two hundred and fifty of us at the present moment has consumption; but at least one adult in every seven of us is going to die of it. All because of this nefarious, wait-till-you're-ill system, which no one has the courage to attack, and because we will not send doctors out to the highways and byways to find disease, and haul it apart so that they may stand between the healthy and the infected and the plague be stayed.

As it is with consumption, so it is with a hundred and one other diseased conditions. Instead of having our doctors come to us while we are well, or think we are well, we refuse to go to them until we are certainly ill, and then we too often learn we have come too late.

As one more instance there may be quoted cancer in women. Here the details are not suitable for placing before lay readers, but it may be pointed out that in the earlier stages, where the surgeon could do something, there is often no pain. There is only what appears to be a harmless swelling, often coming on so slowly that it is hardly noticed, and the patient

E

is not alarmed, or has some false modesty in going to a physician. Later, when the thing becomes more troublesome, she goes, alas, too often to be told, it is too late.

Now, suppose we had established firmly that the only right principle in such cases is an early medical consultation ; and suppose, further that which is essential for the majority of case; occurring amongst poor working women or the wives of workmen, that we had established such a National Medical Service that this consultation could be obtained gratis, and as thorough and skilful as if the individual patient were paying for it, and, most important of all, without having to lose practically a day's work going to the Out-patient Department of a Charity Hospital. What a change this would make, what a revolution in our whole system ; how many useful lives might be spared, and homes left bright on which death now casts its shadow !

CHAPTER IV

OUR HOSPITAL SYSTEMS: THEIR EVILS AND ABUSES

THERE is no virtue so well-beloved as charity, nor any to which so many counterfeits of all kinds exist, so closely resembling the real article that it is often difficult to expose the fraud.

But just as matter in the wrong place is dirt, so the most admirable virtue turned from its right use becomes vice.

A sincere and practical commiseration for the woes of our fellow-men leading to well-directed acts of charity or benevolence, whether given in service or in money, must always excite the admiration of the noble-minded.

It is for this reason that the sentiment and lofty purpose which have founded and maintained our Voluntary Hospital system have received so much admiration and eulogy for generations.

The author has no fight to wage with such high sentiments as these, and as his own object is the alleviation of human suffering, just as is that of the philanthropist of the voluntary hospital, this common aim and objective must be his excuse for pointing out some of the limitations in our present equipment for reaching our destination, and showing that our energies may perhaps better be turned into another channel of approach.

In the task of destroying disease and abolishing destitution we require, and must have, the aid of every one in the nation who is capable of assisting; there must be no shirking of what is every one's duty, and each must be eager to do his share.

The contribution to be exacted does not always mean money; sometimes it means service, skill, privation, or separation. The demands of disease-fighting are inexorable; there is no royal path for any one; disease is no respecter of persons or conditions; we must fight it in a scientific way, or we must suffer defeat. A few lunatics, or ignoramuses, with conscientious objections, or some other form of lunacy such as faith-healing, can wreck our whole scheme, so that it cannot be voluntary; it can only succeed when the voice of the majority of the people demands it and it is backed by a strong Government.

Now, in spite of all its lofty sentiments of voluntary charity and benevolence, the curse of the voluntary hospital system—and it is a great curse—is that it is blinding the eyes of those who could most help social reform to the fact that we possess no National Hospital System. The Voluntary System is utterly inadequate; it is strained to its utmost limit and almost bankrupt, and yet it cannot attend to more than about fifteen to twenty per cent. of the cases requiring attention. By its very excellence in attending to this small proportion of the suffering poor, it blinds our eyes and blunts our perceptions in regard to the eighty per cent. which it does not touch at all.

This is the keynote, the fundamental failure, in our hospital system, and must not be lost sight of in any detailed description of other hospital evils and abuses which follow in this chapter.

A system which cannot do more than fifteen per cent., or twenty at the outside, of the work which it is intended to do, and this after generations of highest effort, is a hopeless failure, and is a vice and a drawback, because it stands in the way of the introduction of a proper organised scientific effort.

Even this small proportion of work done by the Voluntary Hospitals is by no means perfect, nor is it uniform in its standard throughout the country; but even if it were perfect, how by voluntary effort is it to be made to extend to deal with the eighty per cent. at least of work which is now either done most execrably by the Poor Law Authorities, or left undone altogether?

The best and warmest friends of the voluntary system must admit that any such five- or six-fold extension is utterly impossible, and out of the question.

Now, from personal experience and examination, the author vouches that the poor persons in the Voluntary Hospitals differ in no way or respect from the poor persons in the Poor Law Hospitals, and these again from those helpless in the slums unable to obtain admission to either type of hospital.

If this be so—and it will be hard to controvert it—the whole position is illogical and utterly untenable to any thinking person.

Further, it may be truly said that any person who contributes towards or endows voluntary hospitals, however good his or her intentions, is contributing to the perpetuation of a great national nuisance and great national wrong which cries aloud for redress.

Such contributions indicate no true charity, but its exact opposite; there is no health in the puling sentimentality which short-sightedly relieves the case in view and wilfully neglects the nine cases, equally deserving, clamouring for attention just around the corner. Such sentimentality, by casting a spurious air of decency about the proceedings, prevents that wholesome exposure which public morality and good faith with ourselves demand.

This is a public sore and festering spot, not to be plastered over with anodynes and ointments till it is hidden from view, and kept out of sight by repeated coatings of the ointment of spurious charity; the sore needs to be opened by the surgeon's knife and treated in a scientific way so that it may be healed, instead of remaining with us for ever.

Let us stop dropping feeble sentimental tears over the sufferings of the poor and doling out charity to them; let us put them under a system which will end these sufferings.

In this process the first essential is the reduction of disease, and for this we must have a unified, organised system of hospitals under the direction and control of our National Medical Service.

Do not turn away and say the Nation cannot afford it, for it is going to cost less by half than our present extravagant and wasteful systems of (1) Voluntary Hospitals, (2) Poor Law Hospitals, (3) Municipal Hospitals, (4) Special Hospitals, (5) Municipal Dispensaries, and, last and worst of all, (6) No Hospitals. Give us one organised system in true co-ordination, instead of all this chaos, and one may venture to guarantee that both disease and expense will drop to one-half together.

In writing with some feeling on these evils of our present hospital systems, the author is not being carried away by imagined horrors, or dealing with matters of which he has heard from another; he has actually seen and experienced these things, and can state as an eye-witness that there is no greater mass of incongruity and absurdity and wasteful extravagance existing anywhere in all the whole fabric of our civilised institutions than the

British Hospitals taken as a whole. Such contrasts of good and evil, light and shade, sanitation and insanitation, order and disorder, wealth of space and overcrowding, highest medical skill and practically no medical attendance, can nowhere be found in such profusion as in the wards of our hospitals.

Let any one who thinks this is the personal view of a crank go and pay a visit to one of our better-class Voluntary Hospitals, and then visit one of our older Poor Law Hospitals, or read, if this is not feasible, the account of the recent Royal Poor Law Commission, both Majority and Minority, as to how the poor are treated in our Poor Law Hospitals.

Those who cannot do this may learn much by consulting the accounts of various hospital inspections throughout the country made by Sir Henry Burdett, K.C.B., and published in the *Hospital* during 1909–10.

There are no arguments so telling as baldly stated facts from concrete instances, so one may contrast here two hospitals existing almost side by side in the same city, the one a Voluntary Charity Hospital and the other a Poor Law Hospital.

Since these two hospitals are but a type of what exists, neither better nor worse, over the greater part of the country, and as the object is to describe existing conditions without attaching either praise or blame to administrators, the city and the two hospitals are described under assumed names.

The statements made, however, are mainly based on the author's own personal observations of two actual institutions; and, further, they are substantially in accord with the reports of one of the greatest hospital authorities in the world, on these two institutions.

The two hospitals in question are the Royal Charity Infirmary, Cottonport, and the Guardian Angel Workhouse Infirmary, Cottonport.

The Royal Charity Infirmary contains just under 300 beds, and the Guardian Angel Infirmary contains close on 1000 beds. The 300 patients of the "Royal Charity," in addition to the Consulting Staff, have three visiting physicians and three visiting surgeons to investigate and attend to their illnesses, while over 900 patients at the "Guardian Angel" have one visiting physician and one visiting surgeon to perform a like office. There is a Gynæcological Surgeon and an Assistant Gynæcological Surgeon, with a resident House Surgeon under them, to attend to gynæcological cases at the Royal Charity Infirmary; in the more than three times larger Guardian Angel Infirmary there is no gynæcologist, all gynæcological operations being performed by the single visiting surgeon. There are at the Royal Charity Infirmary an ophthalmic surgeon, a laryngologist, a dermatologist, a surgeon in charge of the X-Ray Department, and four medically qualified Anæsthetists—there are no such officers at the more than threefold larger Guardian Angel Infirmary, only a few hundred yards distant in the same city of Cottonport.

There are, in addition to the Senior Honorary Staff of the Royal Charity Infirmary, three Hon. Assistant Surgeons and two Hon. Assistant Physicians; there is no corresponding staff whatever at the Guardian Angel Infirmary. There are a medical registrar, a surgical registrar, three house physicians, and five house surgeons to look after the 300 patients at the Royal Charity Infirmary, while there are four resident medical officers all told at the Guardian Angel Infirmary to attend to nearly 1000 patients.

Summing up these facts, there are *twenty-one* Visiting Medical Officers attached to the Royal Charity Infirmary, and *ten* Resident Medical Officers; while there are *two* Visiting Medical Officers and *four* Resident Medical Officers at the Guardian Angel Infirmary; and it may be finally reiterated that the former institution has less than 300 beds, and the latter well over 900 beds.

So much for the relative Staffs of the two Hospitals: now as to equipment. The Royal Charity Infirmary is modern and up-to-date, while the Guardian Angel Infirmary is antiquated, and in the opinion of many competent authorities, ought to have been pulled down years ago. The buildings for the 300 patients cost at least double as much as those for the

1000 patients. It is difficult, without actual
measurements, to estimate relative air-spaces,
but there is quite double, probably treble, as
much air-space per patient at the Royal Charity
Infirmary as at the Guardian Angel Infirmary.

The sanitary arrangements at the " Guardian
Angel" scarcely can bear description. There are
only *two* baths, pre-Roman in their appearance,
for each floor of one hundred and fifty beds,
and these two baths have to be used for such
washing purposes, as well as the patients' bodies,
which exigency requires to be done upon the
spot—such, for example, as the soiled waterproof
sheets from the beds. The common closets, in
an open row, and the common latrine on each
floor, "beggars all description," but not for the
same reason as Cleopatra in her barge, although
here also "a strange invisible perfume hits the
sense."

In contrast, the sanitary arrangements at the
"Royal Charity" are all that the requirements
of a modern hospital demand. Each ward
possesses its own set of (1) patients' wash-up
room, (2) bathroom, (3) set of separated closets,
and (4) nurses' sanitary wash-out room with air-
shaft to outer air. This set of four sanitary
rooms is built apart from the main ward in a
Sanitary Tower separated from the ward by a
well-ventilated vestibule. The whole system is
walled by glazed fireclay brick, easily kept in
clean condition.

In the wards themselves, the floors at the

" Royal Charity " are of oak parquetry, while at the " Guardian Angel " they are of common deal, cracked, splintered, seamed, and worn everywhere till the many knots stand up like the gnarled excrescences of a gouty old age. The walls are of glazed brick at the " Royal Charity "; at the " Guardian Angel " they are roughly plastered and painted over.

Attached to each ward of the " Royal Charity," these wards containing eighteen to thirty-two beds only, there are the following working accessories: (1) a small isolation ward containing two beds, and (2) a convalescent room for patients able to walk about. To every two wards there is a small clinical laboratory assigned, in which chemical and bacteriological investigations and other scientific examinations relating to the cases can be carried out, and these laboratories are well fitted with scientific appliances. No slightest vestige of these up-to-date requirements exist at the " Guardian Angel," where there is no means for examination or investigation in the whole vast institution.

One surgeon only, the visiting surgeon, has hitherto performed all the surgical operations deemed necessary for the whole of the patients of this huge hospital (" Guardian Angel "), including all the gynæcological cases. For all these operations there are provided only two *small* surgical theatres situated in attics on two top floors, one for the male hospitals and one for the female hospitals. In each of these divisions there are over 400 beds, probably half of which are surgical—that is to say, there is one little, antiquated theatre for a hospital of over 400 beds, and one *half* the services of a single visiting surgeon.

The patients at the "Guardian Angel" are anæsthetised in the operating theatre itself, and when one thinks of the demands on one operating surgeon's time in such a huge institution, it is probable that a previous patient is usually undergoing an operation when the next is carried into the operating theatre *on stretchers*. There is no passenger lift to the whole of each huge four-storied block (or, rather, three blocks arranged in the worst possible manner and buttressed up by other buildings), and hence the unfortunate patients have to be carried to and from the operating theatre on stretchers along narrow corridors and up and down steep and awkward stone staircases. It suggests forcibly to one's mind certain adaptations of the lines on the pauper's burial by Tom Hood.[1]

There is no steam steriliser in either of these two small theatres; there are two operating tables in each, of a most antique gridiron pattern, quite unadaptable for the different surgical positions; the floor is of common boards, the furnishings of the most parsimonious character,

[1] Such as :—

> Rattle his stretcher up and down stairs ;
> He's only a pauper, and nobody cares.

and the instruments scanty and often out-of-date.

On the other hand, the "Royal Charity" possesses four large operating theatres, each replete with all modern conveniences, with anæsthetising rooms attached to each; and there are two commodious hydraulic lifts from floor to floor, and rubber-tyred trolley couches on which the patients are conveyed to and from the wards and operating theatres.

With such a Staff as we have seen is provided at the "Guardian Angel," it goes without saying that there cannot be much order or arrangement of the patients in the wards, or adequate note-taking or attention to the progress of the cases. On account of an ingenious space-saving device of the architect, who probably flourished and was gone before the science of bacteriology had made much progress, it comes to pass that the ends of several of the wards are veritable boxes, having quite blank walls without windows on three sides for at least half their length, and on the day of the writer's visit there were phthisical and non-phthisical patients lying side by side on beds not very wide apart in these window-less ends of wards.

There was a considerable number of such phthisical patients, and it was explained to me by my conductor that these patients were mixed up with the others *because the phthisis wards were full.*

Two special wards for phthisis on the male side, and one on the female side, each with low-pitched roof, had no windows whatever to the open air on three of their walls, and the few windows on the one free side were small and high. Two of the walls were quite devoid of windows; the third had borrowed light and air from a long, dark corridor running between this ward and a fellow ward in a parallel tier with it. But this poor corridor had little of air and less of light for the wards to borrow from it.

Just reflect on the above, *as a ward for phthisical cases*, in the year of grace, nineteen hundred and ten.

When the press of phthisical cases becomes too great, the more convalescent patients, it appears, are sometimes sent over to the general workhouse.[1] A visit to one of the bedrooms of this place revealed in a room little better than a cellar, with windows on two adjacent sides only, *and these all tightly closed*, about forty men in beds packed closely together. The atmosphere was vile and heavy at 9 P.M.; its condition from midnight till morning can be left to the imagination. Is it wonderful, when tuberculosis is so carefully cultivated in our midst, that our national death-roll from this plague runs up to 75,000 annually?

---

[1] This statement does not rest on the author's own personal observation, but on information volunteered by an officer of the institution.

To go on painting the comparative details of the "Royal Charity" and "Guardian Angel" Hospitals would only be to become wearisome; no high colouring, no embellishment, is necessary.

In these two hospitals, then, within a stone's-throw of each other in the same city, we find this obvious contrast. Both contain only poor people unable to pay for medical treatment, for that is the reiterated guarantee of all the Charity Hospitals, that they admit no one who can afford to pay; and indeed, under present conditions, that is only very elementary justice to the medical profession outside. Also, apart from ability to pay, there is no moral distinction of any kind between the two sets of patients. Examine the causes of disease in each institution if you are a medical man, and you may notice the same diseases, due to the same causes, in the one institution as in the other. In the Poor Law Institution, on the occasion of one's visit, one saw several old veterans who had served their country well in the Crimean campaign and later wars; respectable old chaps they seemed to be, who only had come upon dark days in their old age.

There is not a thing, not a point of difference, between the two sets of patients, and hence the irresistible question arises, Why is one set treated so well, and the other set—over three times as large, be it remembered—treated so badly?

Both ways of it cannot be right; if the "Royal Charity" treatment is the proper one to accord to poor people who cannot pay for themselves when they are ill, then we are behaving with austerity, to use a mild term, to the inmates of the "Guardian Angel." Contrariwise, if the "Guardian Angel" treatment indicates the proper way, then we are pampering the inmates of the "Royal Charity."

There is no attempt here to attach either praise or blame to the two sets of people who administer these two institutions. Could every circumstance be taken into account, the Poor Law Guardians of the "Guardian Angel" might be found to have been doing as admirable a work under highly adverse conditions of environment as the better-circumstanced Committee of the "Royal Charity." That is not the question for us here at all; there is no personal element in the matter—it is a matter of principle purely and simply. We require a unified, co-ordinated system of treating in hospital those large numbers who are unable to pay, and this picture, in contrasts, is intended to illustrate how far we are from having any such system at present.

Surely we ought to make some attempt to arrive at some principle of even-handed justice in these matters.

It might possibly be argued that although there is no difference in poverty or deserts between the two sets of patients, there is a difference in the relationships of the two insti-

F

tutions to the community, in that the "Royal Charity" is a great teaching hospital, where our future doctors are trained, and where medical science is advanced, and new discoveries made of great advantage to all mankind. To this there are two obvious replies which at once rob the argument of all significance. In the first place, all this greater comfort in the Voluntary Hospital is not necessary for the study of disease ; and, secondly, there is no reason, except a most stupid and arbitrary law or rule of the Local Government Board, why the Poor Law Hospitals should not be used for medical study, instruction, and research.

A teacher of clinical medicine or surgery at a medical school would find the wealth of clinical material of Guardian Angel Poor Law Hospital, and its value for teaching, as great as that of any Voluntary Hospital in the Country.

Why is this vast store of rich clinical material in our University towns throughout the country absolutely thrown away and wasted ? Can the country afford to have any but the best of clinical experience placed at the disposal of the future doctors ?

Are the officials of the Local Government Board afraid of the susceptibilities of the poor patients in the hospitals under their purview, that they absolutely forbid entry for medical study, both to the medical student and the practitioner of the district ? Or is it perchance that the Boards of Guardians are afraid to press home the Local Government Board to grant this boon for their districts?

It cannot surely be the susceptibilities of the pauper patients, for that cannot be greater than that of the patients in the Voluntary Hospitals, who are equally accepting charity there.   No; we must look for some other cause for this strange order of things, this subtle distinction between the recipients of Poor Law Charity and the recipients of Voluntary Charity, which makes the diseases of the latter worthy of study, while those of the former are beneath contempt, let alone study.

Is it perhaps because the officials think the diseases of paupers are quite different from those of other people?   If so, they might at least appoint a Royal Commission to inquire into the matter, and then consider both Minority and Majority Report, and pigeon-hole the results for their successors in office.

It cannot surely be because the honorary physicians and surgeons of the great teaching hospitals, those great guns of the profession, would feel their craft in danger were any *common* doctor at a Poor Law Hospital allowed to teach from the clinical material at his disposal, and that too great access to clinical material might open too many gateways to knowledge?   No! perish the thought.

The brightest thoughts always come last, and the most probable thing dawns on one when the problem seems hopeless of solution.   How could the present-day methods of treating Poor Law patients stand the free ingress of batches of fresh young students, free to see and to talk publicly outside of what they saw inside? Just about as much as the hot-house plants of a conservatory could stand the cold breath of the winter winds. There would be too much moral ventilation about letting medical students into workhouse hospitals; these institutions contain much that is best hidden from the light, and the medical student is a bit of a reformer, and an irresponsible enthusiast for justice.

Open the gates of the workhouse infirmaries to the public, and the medical student who will bring the public in after him, and the whole system is exploded; it will not last out even a single parliament.

If the Poor Law Authorities only admitted medical students to their hospitals, the Poor Law medical appointments would at once rise in value to members of the medical profession; these posts could soon be filled by the best physicians and surgeons in all our large cities, where there are universities and medical schools, and the filling of them need not cost the Guardians a penny. The physicians and surgeons who aspired to be consultants would be tripping over one another to get appointed.

This is merely pointed out as a suggestion to the proper public authorities who may want to save money; in the opinion of many sound judges, the system of paying a would-be consul-

tant by bringing him into contact with students
is a most abominable practice. Every official
of a hospital should be paid for his duties
properly in salary, and there ought to be so
many such appointments that any man's position as a consultant came to depend on his
real skill and knowledge, and not upon his
hanging on to a hospital and getting to know
and be known of students.

Returning to our contrast of the Voluntary
and Poor Law Hospital systems, we may now
attempt to answer the oft-made criticism, why,
if the Voluntary Hospitals are so much better,
and many of the Poor Law Hospitals are so
wretched, suggest the abolition of the Voluntary system, and the substitution of a Public
or State system, since a public system under
the Poor Law is doing so badly? The two
hospitals just described might surely be taken
as illustrating the advantages of a voluntary
system over a publicly controlled system. The
answer is that the Voluntary system is like an
exotic plant which cannot be made to flourish
sufficiently so that it may grow at least six-
fold as large and do all the work, and meanwhile, by the place it occupies in the public
eye, it glozes over and palliates a great evil.

By all means let us keep our Voluntary Hospitals for the present, if only we can remember
that they are not solving a great national question
which is pressing urgently for solution.

Let us go on, if we must, playing at Charity

like children with their toys in a nursery, if only at times we will come out of the land of make-believe and see that we are not really doing what we pretend we are doing.

As for the Poor Law Hospital system, that is a failure, not because it is under a public system of administration, but because that system is so wretchedly devised, and has been going on upon wrong principles year after year for three generations. Under the Poor Law it is a shocking disgrace, for which, till just recently, your enlightened country disfranchised you, to be poor and in ill-health. It is necessary that the pauper patient should be treated just as horridly and uncomfortably as our twentieth-century state of decency of public feeling can permit, in order that the poor sick person shall not go to the Workhouse Infirmary to be a charge on the rates until the last gasp, or until poor suffering human nature can save its public degradation no longer, and crawls, or is carried by the police, into the Workhouse Hospital to die.

It is a well-deserved penalty upon us that in this cheese-paring attempt to spare our pockets we save neither them nor our consciences nor reputations, but all suffer together. The few millions we *seem* to save in this way are ten-fold outbalanced by the cost borne by us on account of disease rampant over the country through the operation of this very system.

We think, or our Boards of Guardians think

for us, that a public service has been done when one junior medical man has been paid £120 to £150 a year to pretend he is properly looking after four to five hundred beds filled with sick people in a Workhouse Hospital, and no medical officer at all is sent out to the slums to send the rest of them into the hospital, where, if it were properly organised, they ought to be receiving proper attention. But is it so? In very truth we pay tenfold in cash alone for our sin of inhumanity, not to mention that upon which no value in money can ever be put, the sacrifice of those dear to us as life itself carried off by the infections cultured in workhouse and slumland.

The second great count which may be made in this indictment of our present miscellaneous congeries of hospital systems is that they are hopelessly out of touch with the medical practitioners throughout the country, and that this is most highly detrimental alike to the public service, to the hospitals themselves, and to the medical profession.

Any layman who may think this statement is too sweeping may be invited to make inquiries amongst two or three of his medical acquaintances, and, especially if he happens to ask a doctor who has any practice amongst working people, as most doctors have, he will very rapidly be satisfied as to the true position of affairs as between hospitals and the profession.

If he will ask the one question, "Dr. So-and-so, what is the meaning of this hospital abuse that we hear spoken of occasionally?" he need say no more; he will have waved the proverbial "red rag," or "touched the button," if you prefer the simile, and "the doctor will do the rest." Just try the experiment the next time you happen to meet a genuine general medical practitioner; it is guaranteed to succeed nine times, at least, out of every ten.

So it would with you, my dear reader, whatever your profession or business may happen to be, if some one were trying to oust you out of it and do your work for nothing by means of a so-called charity subscribed by other people.

Suppose that three-quarters at least of your income came to you from a certain set of clients, as three-fourths of the average medical practitioner's income does to him from the wage-earning classes, and that a large number of very benevolent people subscribed to set up institutions to perform the work for these clients that you had been doing before, and that on account of the charitable subscriptions and the conspiracy of a number of your colleagues in your own profession, this work, previously paid for to you, was now done gratuitously, and without recouping you in any shape or form, so that your income started to dwindle as your clients gradually discovered this new method of satisfying their wants.

Now, one may ask, supposing you were

gifted with an average human temper, what
would you think of all this, and in what
language would you clothe your thoughts (1)
as to the charitable people, (2) as to the institutions, and (3) as to your colleagues in the
institutions who did your work for nothing?

Perhaps some consideration of your answers
to these questions may mellow your opinions
of the doctor who has replied to your query as
to what is "hospital abuse," and if one tells
you further that, in spite of his chafed feelings,
the doctor so far forgives the colleague who
does his work for nothing in the hospital
that he throws highly paid work in his way
with assiduity, and takes him out to see his
wealthier patients to earn large fees from them,
as a consultant and a brother, you will probably
grow to regard the general medical practitioner
as an exemplary prototype of a charitable
Christian gentleman, or—something else.

In both cases you will be quite wrong; the
general medical practitioner may be both these
things, but that does not explain his peculiar
conduct. As a matter of fact, both he and
his hospital colleague, the consultant, are in
the grip of a vicious circle.

There is only one way out, and that is a
State Medical Service, and State Hospitals for
all members of the wage-earning classes.

Such a system gives co-ordination between
medical attendance on the wage-earners outside,
and medical and surgical attendance for them

within the hospitals. As a result hospital abuse is done away with, because it simply cannot exist, and the doctor, whether his work lies within or without the hospital, is adequately recompensed for his labour.

For the serious surgical diseases and injuries amongst the wage-earning classes, hospitals are absolutely indispensable. Major surgical operations cannot be carried out efficiently and safely in the cottages of the poor, and even in the middle and upper-middle classes it is becoming increasingly recognised that surgical operations and careful nursing are best carried out in a special institution such as the private paying ward of a hospital or a nursing-home. The working classes used to dread a hospital operation and preferred to pay their doctor and have it done at home, but this feeling is rapidly passing away, and in a few years will be non-existent. The change is due to many factors, such as (1) the action of medical practitioners themselves in sending poor patients to hospital because they honestly cannot contemplate carrying through a serious operation and after-nursing at the patient's own home, or, in other cases, see that the patient cannot pay for such prolonged attendance and nursing; (2) the much-decreased mortality, under modern conditions, of surgical operations in hospitals as compared with private houses, especially amongst the poorer classes, and the better equipment and conditions of living in the voluntary hospitals making the patient's sojourn there much more comfortable than a few years ago; (3) the excessive cost of a surgical operation at home, even amongst the middle classes; (4) the growing feeling that an institution which is supported in so many diverse ways, and to which even the workmen, by weekly contributions and Saturday and Sunday collections, yield their quota, is no longer a charity, but an institution to which all have almost the right of entry when there is room and they have need.

When Voluntary Hospitals were first instituted, and indeed to within a decade or so ago, it was on the assumption that they were for the relief of the poor, meaning thereby the very poor of the labouring class; but developments have been such, both in scientific medicine and surgery, and in our general public point of view with regard to hospitals, that the voluntary hospitals are now generally regarded as open to nearly all of the wage-earning class up to, at any rate, a wage-earning power of two pounds a week. Even a man earning three pounds a week will not be denied admittance for a serious surgical operation, although he may be expected to make some small contribution to the hospital funds.

This state of affairs is most deplorable so long as the relationships of private practitioner and hospital remain unadjusted, and, by setting up the practitioner and hospital as rivals, is responsible for that hatred and excitement throughout the profession which is almost producing a condition of war between the profession and the hospitals. This condition is the inevitable result of the specialisation in surgical work which has arisen, and of the inordinately high fees which surgeons are compelled to charge for work done outside the hospital. A surgeon nowadays can make quite a comfortable income on one good operation a week, which perhaps occupies no more than a couple of hours of his time all told; and a busy surgeon with a fast motor-car can make a princely income. Nor does he usually possess any of that genius for craftsmanship, or advanced knowledge of science, which might reasonably be expected to carry such a huge income as its reward.

He may in intellect and ability be nothing like so fine a man as his poorer colleague in medicine, or the medical scientist who plods along upon an income of five or six hundred a year, after previous years of struggle and poverty.

His art is almost purely mechanical, and even at that often does not require exceptional manipulative ability. The secret of the situation is that he belongs to a small close craft with a very limited *entrée* to its ranks, and a path of some expense, anxiety, and delay at the outset.

The distinguished hospital surgeon is often a man of very mediocre attainments, whom years of practice on certain lines of work has placed

in a unique position. He has shown keenness
and patience, and trained his hands well to
manipulation, but often he has not added one
line, or precept, or practical application to the
craft of which he is an exponent. He has
usually taken for his hobby the acquirement of
guineas, a bias acquired in those years of waiting and difficulty when the golden ones came
in but slowly. His boast is that he makes
more than his rival, Mr. So-and-so; not, alas,
too often, that he has done anything to adorn
the Science and Art of Surgery.

His period of large income making is a shorter
one than that of the physician, for after twenty
years of golden harvests his palmiest days are
over.

It is a sad thing, both for the public interests
and for surgical science itself, that it should be
so converted into an article of commerce.

The evil concerns more than the wage-earning classes; middle-class people with incomes of
the range of, say, £400 to £800 are also hardly
hit by this grotesque arrangement which renders
it impossible for more than about one medical
man in fifty to carry through successfully a
quite straightforward surgical operation.

The middle-class or professional business man
has to pay the penalty when he requires to submit
to a surgical operation, either upon himself or
some member of his family. He has then to
help to pay for all those cases which the surgeon
has been doing for nothing at the hospital, and

has the defects of this system brought home to him, although he may hardly know what has hit him.   He may wonder in a vague way why the highest possible surgical technique is *always* required, and he has to pay £50 to £100 for it, in addition to all the incidental expenses of preparation and nursing.   He might be horrified, poor man, if he were told that the same thing was done in hospital every day for nothing; and if he had enough knowledge to appreciate a visit to a modern hospital operating-room and surgical ward, might realise that his operation could have been carried out better there, surrounded by all the appliances and accessories of the Art of Surgery, than in his suburban villa, to which the surgeon hurriedly brings such things as he thinks or foresees he may want in his hand-bag. All the upset to his household and family, too, might be spared, and his chances of recovery would brighten in purely professional hands of surgeon, doctor, and nurse.

There is little or nothing in the way of intermediate grades between the patient who can, or is compelled to, pay much too handsomely and the patient who cannot meet these terms and is forced to be operated upon in hospital for nothing.   Therein lies half the hospital abuse on the surgical side in our hospitals; and the surgical side is twice as great as the medical.

Another great danger to a certain middle class of patients is the very natural jealousy of the hospital engendered in the mind of the practitioner by this process of robbing him of his patients. His fees all stop when the patient goes to hospital. Is it natural, therefore, that even when he knows that all the circumstances of the case demand an operation, which can only properly be carried out in a hospital, that he will be prompt to urge his patient to go to hospital without delay?

There are very many cases, on the surgical side especially, in which palliative treatment can be pursued for a long time with varying chances of success, continually putting off the evil day, a process to which the patient is only too prone to listen with favour. Here commences a struggle between the practitioner's purse and his conscience; to the honour of the profession, be it said, that conscience usually wins; but why should he be subjected to any such struggle, with his feelings already at white heat against the hospitals?

The practitioner is hopelessly handicapped in the struggle: all the accessories of the scene are against him. He cannot afford to own privately all the instruments and outfit necessary for proper equipment, or provide the staff of assistants required. He has no right of admission as an operator to the well-equipped operating theatre at the hospital, so that he himself can operate, nor can he apply after-treatment in the hospital. His patient is not allowed by the regulations to pay a reasonable fee, and remaining under his own physician's care, who knows all about him, have a specialist to do the operation in the hospital, and then pass back to the care of his own doctor, still in the hospital.

In fact, unless the patient can pay like a very wealthy person, he must be treated like a pauper, and his physician as a nonentity.

In this struggle, which is ever becoming more acute and bitter, of practitioner *versus* hospital, lives of patients are doubtless often lost, for one of two reasons—first, that the patient is sent to the hospital too late; and secondly, that practitioners often operate at patients' homes under unjustifiable conditions, either as to surroundings and means of care and nursing, or as to their own skill as operators. How frequently such instances occur it would be difficult to estimate, but the writer himself, in quite a limited experience, has known more than one clear instance of this danger to the public.

There is another aspect of hospital work which has still further embittered this question of hospital abuse, and that is the barefaced way in which many of the out-patient departments of our Voluntary Hospitals are used for the purpose of defrauding the medical profession.

Unless the out-patient department is used on a purely consultative basis, for the purpose of giving the opinion of the hospital physician or surgeon on a case where the patient is unable to pay a consulting fee, it becomes a clear usurpation of the professional rights of the practising doctor who advises working-class people and earns his living amongst them.

It will be, of course, understood that we are now discussing the defects of our *present* system; all this confusion would automatically disappear under a combined system of State Medical Officers and State Hospitals; but so long as out-patient departments remain part of a voluntary charitable system, and the outside practitioner earns his living by fees instead of receiving a salary as a State official, then the present intolerable state of affairs will remain not only unchecked, but growing in its proportions, as it rapidly is at present.

It may be said, without the least hesitation, that at the present day there is no business or profession being so crushed by wrongful spoliation and confiscation as is the medical profession; and the irony of it is, that it is all being done in the name of charity and benevolence.

If these would-be benefactors of their race would open their eyes to the fact that they are crushing out of existence one of the most humanitarian of all professions, and try to devise some plan on common-sense lines for its rehabilitation and proper recompense, they would do a great service not only to the medical profession but to the poor whom they are desirous of assisting.

It might be some small compensation if the poor were really benefited by this out-patient

G

system, or if medical science were advanced by it, but the exact reverse of all this is the case.

There are two disgraces on the fair name and reputation of medical science to-day, which do more than anything else to reduce medicine to a pseudo-science and trail it through the gutter of contempt in the eyes of all scientists, and those two disgraces are the Out-patient Departments of our Hospitals, and the Sixpenny Dispensary Practice of our Slums. There is not a pin to choose between them as they at present exist, and the sooner they are either remodelled on scientific lines or swept off the fair face of Creation, the better for mankind and our sense of decency.

In both cases the times given are utterly inadequate for proper examination, care, or attention to the cases; as for scientific study of them, or getting to know the habits and constitution of the patient, there is no attempt at such things.

Think first of the absence of all the principles of sanitation in crowding a score or more of people at a given dispensary hour into the front room of a £20 to £30 house; to be hailed out one after another at intervals into the consulting room, hastily catechised, hurriedly examined, given a bottle of medicine and sent away, after collecting the sixpence, to come back in a few days for another bottle of medicine. Think of the fate of the phthisical patient coming there habitually till he gets sick of

it, and sad for it, paying his sixpence and
getting sent back to infect others in his own
home or elsewhere; with no help save his
useless bottle of cough mixture. Think further
of the danger to the score or so of people,
including several children probably, who have
sat for perhaps an hour with that phthisical
patient in that close, overcrowded, stuffy room
waiting for their golden couple of minutes
with the doctor. Think of the poor children
brought there affecting one another with infectious diseases as they sit.

Was there ever such a mad scheme as placing
unexamined diseased people cheek by jowl, and as
closely packed as possible, for an hour or more?

Look next at the out-patient department of
a big hospital and see a similar picture. It is
true much money from the charitable may have
been spent on glazed brick walls and encaustic
tiles, and many of our new out-patient departments look most beautiful and gaudy; but
the tide of filth and infection passing through
them is enormous, and after all a sewer is only
a sewer, even if it be lined with glazed brick.

There they sit, oppressed with various ills,
or with small children ill with different com-
plaints, gossiping with one another by the hour,
or looking utterly bored and dull, thinking
perhaps of their husband's comments when he
comes home from his work and finds no meal
cooked for him. No doctor outside has hitherto
seen them or their children, in all probability,

or only some sixpenny quack such as we have been describing; no one knows what disease they are harbouring, or whether there is anything but curiosity the matter with them at all. An ill-assorted selection they are of the rag-tag and bobtail of humanity. Suddenly the house physician or surgeon appears on the scene, attended by the three or four medical students who are his clerks or dressers, glad to escape from the boredom of attendance at the visit of the honorary physician or surgeon to the in-patients in the wards. Gaily these acolytes of the temple of Medicine scamper through the out-patients who have been waiting the better part of the morning, for it is getting near lunch-time, and in twenty minutes or half-an-hour the motley crowd of the morning is dispersed. A few who are thought to be more serious, or more interesting, are given cards to see an Assistant Physician or Surgeon to out-patients at the attendance-hour in the afternoon, and return to waste more time there, perhaps a whole afternoon; but the majority are packed off as rapidly as possible, with their medicine or dressings repeated for another week or fortnight; and this, forsooth, is competent medical attention.[1]

To these poor people all who see them are

---

[1] The mode of dealing with out-patients differs somewhat at different hospitals; the above sketch is from the personal observation and experience of the author at two great teaching hospitals.

doctors, though twice out of thrice they are seen
by a clerk or dresser, and, perhaps, just as well
attended to as if the rapid glance or shadow of
a qualified man had fallen upon them. The
usual crime of the out-patient department is
the crime of the sixpenny dispensary—want
of individual care and attention, scamping of
medical work save for the occasional interesting case, and great wastage of public time, and
danger of spread of infection.

The remedy is quite obvious upon any friendly
co-operative system between the practitioner
outside and the hospital authorities inside.
But without proper co-operation no remedy
is possible. These people must be seen and
attended to somehow, if not in their own interests, or the interests of common humanity,
then in the interests of the other strata of the
community.

The question is, how is it to be done without sacrificing any one's legitimate interests,
and most effectively on behalf of patients and
community?

The system of voluntary charity is both a
failure as regards doing the work, and defrauds
the private practitioner of his legitimate sphere
of work and legitimate fee. He has spent, or
had spent for him, a large sum of money (at
least £1000) in acquiring his professional training, and has given five of the best years of his life
to hard study as a student of his profession. It is
by no means fair that he is to be sweated at his

work or cheated out of it altogether. On the other hand, a large share of the required work can only be adequately and properly carried out in hospital, and these people, in the majority of cases, cannot pay for it. Yet the medical profession, either inside or outside the hospital, ought not to be expected to undertake this work for nothing. Charity is charity, business is business, and the doctor has his living to make out of his profession.

The problem, notwithstanding, is not an insoluble one, provided we can only be content to leave charity out of it. Let charity tackle a problem of the right dimensions for its successful accomplishment, in doing extraneous and accessory things, such as endowing medical research, providing clinical laboratories, endowing research fellowships for young medical men in connection with the hospitals, subsidising the junior posts so that it is possible for men of brilliant mind but without private incomes to reach the higher hospital posts. But let charity leave alone routine work for the million. In the first place, the task is too great for such sums of money as can be so got together; and, in the second place, simply because the thing comes by charity, and not as a legal right to which they themselves, directly or indirectly, have contributed their quota, this charity is a most demoralising influence, inducing servility and destroying any weak moral fibre that may be there, instead of developing and strengthening it. Let our poor come to the hospital as an absolute legal and moral right, without any shadow of patronage or disgrace in it whatever, any more than there is in an old age pension.

But do not leave the patient, or any other lay person for him, to determine when he ought to go to the hospital; that is the business of the doctor outside, and matters must be so arranged that it is not to the personal disadvantage of the doctor to send the patient to the hospital when he thinks the case requires hospital treatment.

This state of affairs can obviously only be attained by arranging, by some unified and national scheme of action, for the doctor to be paid both inside and outside the hospital for professional services rendered to this huge class of our population, and we have already seen that the cost to the nation would not be excessive.

The last defect in the present system of hospital services which need be described is that of the present mode of appointment of medical officers to our hospitals. The method varies somewhat in Voluntary Hospitals and in Poor Law Hospitals respectively, and we shall consider the two systems separately.

The manner and terms of appointment of physicians and surgeons to our Voluntary Hospitals may at first sight seem a trivial subject compared with the more general national issues which have hitherto been considered, but in reality this question lies deep at the root of the whole matter.

Because such appointments are made practically for life—that is to say, subject to retirement at sixty or sixty-five years of age—and as the number of hospital posts is small compared with the number of men qualified to hold them, the majority of men in practice are cut off from the hospitals entirely. Secondly, as the modes of election are by no means calculated for selecting the best men, the service degenerates. Thirdly, in the most important set of all the Voluntary Hospitals—namely, those in which our future doctors obtain their medical and surgical training—the medical school has no voice in the choice of the hospital staffs. To the men holding these appointments, however, the medical school is forced to hand over many of the most important professorships in the Faculty of Medicine, thus stultifying the work of the Faculty and reacting in a most undesirable fashion upon the teaching and advancement of medical knowledge throughout the country.

One great evil arising from lack of training of a sufficient number of good operating surgeons for the service of the country has already been seen in the inordinately high fees claimed for surgical work.

If a considerable number of posts at the voluntary and other hospitals were held for more limited periods, the appointments being made for periods of, say, five years, a working knowledge of surgical technique would be more widely spread in the medical profession. A similar change in the physicianships is also highly desirable, in order to allow more men to keep in living touch with medical progress.

It is not as if the men actually holding the hospital posts were marked off in any way as a special order of medical priesthood by special previous training, greater intellectual endowment, or special genius or aptitude of any sort, from their fellows in general medical practice. Their being where they are is in most cases a matter of accident as our system of election is at present constituted. Our present system makes it essential that our future consultants must work for several years not merely without monetary reward, but under conditions which entail considerable outlay. Brains do not furnish the essential condition of entry to this highest caste of the doctor's profession; quite mediocre ability gets a man there, provided he has money and patience and can wait. Men with brains do sometimes storm this fortress, and, by undergoing great privation, fight their way forward to noble success as consultants and leaders in medical progress. Such men are the very salt of the profession; but, to say the least of it, our present mode of preference to hospital appointments does not encourage such men.

In what manner do we usually choose the best physician or surgeon when there is a

vacancy on the staff of one of our great Voluntary Hospitals?

By hard canvassing of the members of a
lay committee, who themselves usually know
nothing of the relative professional abilities of
the rival candidates, but are swayed by the
facts of the social standing and influence of
the candidate, or the candidate's friends.

Fulsome testimonials as to the candidate's
abilities are got together and printed by each
candidate; these are circulated, along with
verbal embellishments, by each candidate's social
friends amongst the electors, who are nobbled
to vote one way or another by pressure, cajoling,
or beseeching.

We laugh at some of the ways of the Chinese,
and this is *our* way of selecting the men who
are to be leading physicians or surgeons in our
great cities, and mayhap teach medical science
to the coming generation of medical men.

In a certain great provincial city one large
general hospital has an electoral body of *over
one thousand members*, nearly all laymen, who
elect the physicians and surgeons in this way.
At a recent election several gentlemen who
desired the position of surgeon to the hospital had their claims considered by this huge
electorate, and its friends in the city. Without making any criticisms on what the actual
result of the election happened to be, it might
be suggested that a method which would have
worked equally well, and saved enormous trouble

and expense, would have been that of putting all the names of the candidates in a hat and drawing one out.

It may be said that although a lay committee actually has the electoral power, it is swayed in its opinion by the medical staff of the hospital. This happily does occasionally save the situation ; but in a great many cases the medical committee is not allowed any such influence, or is scared of expressing an opinion through fear of alienating or offending powerful laymen.

Another great evil due to our localised systems, especially noticeable in the large Voluntary Hospitals of our great cities and towns, and most intensely of all in those hospitals connected with medical schools, is the continued inbreeding to which we are committed in obtaining our supplies of consultants and teachers of medical science. With few honourable exceptions, we are absolutely forced to depend on local supply, and there is little or no healthy transference from one district to another.

Since the assistant physicians and surgeons, almost automatically, are advanced as vacancies occur to the full physicianships and surgeon-ships, the election to these junior posts is most important. At this stage the juniors have not yet acquired those lucrative practices which fasten their seniors, like limpets or barnacles to rocks, to one city, so that they cannot be transferred when vacancies occur. An offer from Manchester might attract a promising junior

physician or surgeon from Liverpool, or *vice versâ,*
or London might interchange with either of
these two northern cities at this free-swimming,
larval stage in the development of the future
consulting physician or surgeon.

Very often the absence of any chance of
local successions falling in, drives away most
brilliant men, who see no chance in waiting on.
These unlucky individuals have no opportunities
elsewhere. Each hospital and school is a close
corporation. Why are these things so ; why do
not the senior physicians and surgeons tell the
lay Hospital Committee that each post should be
thrown genuinely open to the whole country, and
make it their business, before each election, to
find out the best possible man for the vacancy ?

Possibly there might be something inartistic
in having too many stars of the first order of
magnitude in the same constellation.

Whatever may be the reason, the fact remains, each place has its own little coterie,
and lives in the light of its own little pre-
judices; there is no national correlation, no
cohesion, nothing comparable to anything so
high as the nervous development of the mollusc,
in our whole system of hospitals, or the appointments to all their important posts.

This vicious principle invades even our Universities. Here we see, on the one hand, in the
scientific posts, the stimulating effect on the
men and on the institution of having the whole
nation to select from when a new appointment

is to be made; on the other hand, when we turn to the important chairs of the final studies in the medical faculty, we find no such freedom and no such stimulus. The Universities are practically forced to appoint to important professorships those physicians and surgeons who have been appointed by the local lay committees of the hospitals as members of the hospital staff.

These men need have contributed little or nothing to our knowledge of any branch of medicine or surgery; and indeed, in most cases, as a matter of fact, they have made no such contributions—they have been too busy making guineas instead. Medicine and surgery have become articles of trade and commerce, and the most successful and most highly honoured consultant is he who makes most thousands a year.

Not even in our Universities and seats of medical learning can we stem this tide of the power of the almighty guinea, and show our appreciation of scientific devotion and deserts by appointing men famous for their original work to our University posts.

The important general subjects of the purely medical curriculum are medicine, surgery, midwifery and gynæcology, and therapeutics. To which of these, or any of the special branches of them, can a man be appointed who is not a local consultant in the same city as the University? The candidate may not have contributed one shred to the world's store of knowledge of his subject, yet merely because he is a local man, and has taught the alphabet of medicine to local students—at great profit to himself, be it added, from the consultation fees it has brought him—he is entitled to become the University professor and the local great expert of his subject. Tartarin of Tarascon pales into insignificance before the local glory of the local professor of a medical subject in a provincial University.

Passing by a rapid transition from this sublime subject to the manner of appointment at the Poor Law Hospitals, we find a much simpler and less elaborate scheme.

Roughly speaking, there are two types of Poor Law Hospital Medical Officers. A very transitory whole-time officer, very hard-worked and paid £120 to £150 a year—that is why he is transitory. A very permanent part-time officer, who strongly believes in the axiom that part-time is much less than whole-time, who, for his part-time, is paid from £200 a year upward[1]— that is why he is permanent.

[1] In addition to his position as visitor, the part-time officer usually can pick up such little unconsidered trifles as Vaccination Officer to the Workhouse, and Certifier of Pauper Lunatics. In this way a nominal income of £200 may readily amount to over £500, and the visitor usually contrives to run in addition a lucrative outside practice in his unemployed spare time. This is all according to Cocker, but does it pay the British ratepayer? The writer knows of more than one Poor Law Medical Officer, receiving £500 a year and over, who also has a large private practice and does not devote more than three hours in the day to his Poor Law work The Local Government Board is supposed to inspect the work of these medical officers, and at its doors lies the responsibility, as the Boards of Guardians possess no powers of review or dismissal after one year's service.

The part-time visiting officer is elected by the lay Board of Guardians, the details of election being much the same as set out above for elections in voluntary hospitals. There is usually a spirited competition for such posts, and the candidate after election develops a fervid admiration for the present administration of the Poor Law, and is a thorough believer in Boards of Guardians.

This numerous class of medical men, and a similar body who hold part-time posts to small urban and rural districts as Medical Officers of Health, or as outdoor medical relief Poor Law Officers, or Poor Law Dispensary Officers, are the most violent opponents of any deep-seated changes in the way of reform, and keep pointing out in the press that a little patching and pressing is all that is required.

The whole-time resident medical officers of the Poor Law Hospitals are quite a different set of men, not at all so contented with their lot as their official superiors, nor so impressed with the beneficent influences of our present Poor Law. For one thing, they are younger men, mostly just graduated, and unaccustomed to Workhouse ways, and youth is both sympathetic and fond of change.

Also, they have not time to become truly enamoured of the noble service to which they belong. In entering it they have usually had no thought of continuing in it, as most young men who enter other public services have.

They only want a little more hospital work and experience, and they know that in the Poorhouse Service they can get it in plenty, so they go to it for a brief period of six months to a year, just as they would to a *locum*.

In fact, there is no prospect whatever for young men in this service as a permanency. Their salary never increases, there is no promotion from one place to another, and when a part-time visiting appointment falls vacant they have no claim on it, even if they have been there as resident for ten years.

There is, in fact, no real Poor Law Medical Service; the six hundred and forty odd Poor Law Unions in England and Wales are absolutely independent, have nothing to do with one another, and know no more of one another officially than two next-door neighbours in a London suburb.

The chief products of our Poor Law system, in its hospitals as elsewhere, are disease, demoralisation, and destitution, and those who talk of schemes of reconstruction destroying the moral fibre, self-help, and independence of the poor had better go and visit our Workhouses and learn facts as to the hopeless failure of the present system of repression and mismanagement, when they will probably return prepared to vote for some organised national method for dealing with the greatest national problem of our time.

Until our hospital systems are organised and

unified and placed in *bon accord* with the medical profession outside—the latter having also been nationalised and set to hunt out, isolate, and suppress disease—we may expect to continue to be ravaged by infection. But remember that science has already taught us how most diseases may be conquered, when we are ready to take concerted action for the common weal.

CHAPTER V

THE WARFARE WITH THE GREAT WHITE PLAGUE

A DISEASE which claims seventy-five thousand victims every year, year in, year out, in these Islands of ours alone, is too all-pervading to have escaped incidental mentioning in these pages already. But, when our design is to disclose a feasible, practical method, not of any inordinate cost, whereby this horrible plague can be eradicated in a period of not more than ten years, the subject is assuredly worth a chapter to itself.

When the great bacteriologist who has recently been taken from us, Robert Koch, made the memorable discovery of the bacillus of tuberculosis, and proved that this organism was the one and only cause of the disease known as consumption or phthisis, one of the greatest advances of modern medicine commenced, and one fraught with the highest advantage for mankind.

Diseases rapidly became correlated and understood which before were thought to be quite distinct and separate entities. Consumption was soon realised to be due entirely to the ravages of this organism in the lung substance, a favourite elective seat for its growth in the body, and the same organism growing in the skin was found to be the cause of the dreadfully disfiguring and intractable disease known as lupus. A very common condition, due to decay in the substance of bones, giving rise, according to its situation, to caries of the spine, to hip-joint disease, or to chronic disease of the other joints, was found also to be tuberculosis. A malady, commonest in children, but occurring also in adults, and known as *tabes mesenterica*, or consumption of the bowel, was definitely tracked to its source and again shown to be caused by the same microscopic organism. One common form of a rapidly fatal inflammatory condition of the lining membrane of the brain, known as meningitis, was also traced to that same ubiquitous microbe which Koch's genius had discovered to be the one and only cause of consumption of the lungs.

The changes caused by the growth of this organism vary in appearance to the naked eye, according to the seat of its growth in the body, and this had put off the track earlier pathologists or morbid anatomists, for in those days medical science revolved around anatomy.

Not to go on multiplying examples, we can easily see how this unifying and vivifying discovery cast a flood of light into many dark corners.

The first essential in battling with disease is

to discover the cause of it. It is necessary to know who your enemy is, and where he is, before you can very efficiently strike him; and when you do know that, the next thing is to hit him before he hits you, or is in possession of your fortress. It is not necessary to put a bullet into each of the enemy's soldiers to win the fight; medication which works on this plan too often kills all the friendly soldiers at the same time.

The location of the enemy by Koch's discovery has opened the way to rational methods of attack upon all forms of tubercular disease, making it possible to give sound advice as to treatment and prevention, and it is largely due to this good influence that the death-rate from pulmonary tuberculosis has fallen so much in recent years, that so many less visages are scarred and disfigured by lupus than formerly, and that cripples with stiff and useless joints, curved spines, or absent limbs are so much rarer than before. Conservative surgery, as well as conservative medicine, owes much to Koch's great discovery.

The great disappointment of all the world, and for many hundreds of thousands despair, which followed the failure of Koch's tuberculin as a remedial agent for the individual infected with consumption, dimmed in the eyes of the lay world the lustre of Koch's achievement, and robbed him in the public gaze of that effulgence of glory which ought then to have been, and must henceforward for all time be his, for the discovery of the organism of the disease.

This discovery has already saved hundreds of thousands of lives, and, as the years pass away, will go on saving, and still saving, throughout the coming centuries.

Thanks to Koch, we know, beyond cavil or perchance, that tuberculosis in all its forms is an infectious disease, like smallpox and typhoid and typhus fever, and, like them, can be subjected and held in thrall.

The individual knows now, what he could never be told before, that no one born into this world of ours need die of consumption because his father or mother died from it. In fact, if he is already uninfected, his chance of escape is as good as that of any other individual. There is no immunity against consumption, and, apart from greater chances of infection and want of resistance in the poorer classes, no predisposition has been clearly proven.

As far as the national aspects of the problem are concerned, we are the absolute masters of our own destinies. If we, as a nation, are prepared to take action, there need be no tuberculosis throughout the length and breadth of the land within ten years' time. Any sporadic or chance case turning up after that time can be controlled as easily as we now control smallpox or typhus fever, and we do not even require vaccination of everybody to secure this consummation.

This is no fairy tale, or dream of imagination; it is a definite scientific result, which our present knowledge gives assurance would inevitably follow an equally definite scientific course which is absolutely possible to carry out.

Our training in medicine and methods of studying medical science has given our minds such a bias that it is our most deeply rooted conviction that the first thing we must do is to find a *cure* for each disease. All our study of causation, and our main conceptions as to the use and value of all those sciences allied to medicine, are grouped around this most fundamentally erroneous *dogma* that our main object is to cure disease, and to find out cures at all hazards. We are fundamentally and by nature " medicine men " as assuredly as were witches, charmers, exorcists, and barber-leeches in the old days, and as are all cow-doctors, herbalists, faith-healers, and quack-medicine-vendors in our own days.

The public has been brought up on it all, far more than it has on its mothers' milk, and the medical profession caters for this depraved appetite for drugs and charms, and panders to it everywhere.

The patient wants a drug or a rub; or a plaster or an ointment; or a pill or a powder; or an injection or a snuff; or a gargle or something else; anything to get the disease exorcised out of him. But he will not pay, even in taxes, to have the disease kept away from him; nor take the trouble to avoid it, when he is told how to do so.

How we misread and misapply the lessons of Nature here, in giving all care to the individual and neglecting the species! Nature never does this—her care is for the species; there she is most careful; as to the individual, she is a very prodigal. Would it not be worth while to copy this example, and save the species from tuberculosis by improving the environment?

Only a small percentage of the individuals already attacked can be saved as we work at present; that percentage can be much increased, and in addition infection of new cases can be stopped, if we at once stop working on the individual treatment lines, and start working on species lines.

In order that the tremendous force of this may be felt, it may be reiterated that of the present population of these Islands, not more than one individual in two hundred to three hundred at the present identical moment (as you read this) is suffering from tuberculosis, or need die of tuberculosis; but as we are going on, and unless something is done to arrest it, *one* adult individual out of every *seven* is going to die from tuberculosis.[1]

[1] According to the Decennial Report (1891–1900) of the Registrar-General of Births, Deaths, and Marriages, 1908, Pt. 2, p. xci., eleven per cent. of *all* deaths, or *one* in *nine,* are due to tuberculosis. If allowance be made for our great infantile death-rate, the death-rate from tuberculosis of all adults rises to about one in seven. In males, engaged in occupations, between the ages of fifteen and sixty-five, the rate for consumption alone rises in some trades to over *one* in *three* dying from all causes.

The statement has been made above that the failure of Koch's tuberculin as a treatment caused bitter disappointment. Koch undoubtedly made a mistake by his haste ; all geniuses do make mistakes, and the great German scientist was no exception. That man who has never made a mistake has never done much *in* the World, or *for* the World. *We, also, have all been making mistakes over this tuberculin business;* many unavailing tears have been shed over it ; let us take a different look at the problem.

Had Koch's tuberculin been as great a success as any specific cure in the whole range of modern medicine, tuberculosis would have been just as rampant as it is to-day. One cannot suppress disease by discovering specific cures.

In fact, had Koch's tuberculin been a success, we should probably be suffering now from more prevalence of tuberculosis, simply because we should have still more neglected precautionary and preventive measures than we have done. Let us not pass too hurriedly away from the above remarkable statement, that the discovery of specific remedies will not remove diseases but rather tend to perpetuate them. It sounds like a dangerous heresy, and is therefore worthy of some examination.

Here is another statement more remarkable still :—The possession of a most powerful specific remedy for a given disease, *with our present-day modes of practice and employing it*, may produce little or no effect upon the death-rate from the disease.

If these two statements can be proven to be true, surely it is worth while to discover what is wrong, and if possible right the wrong, otherwise there is little purpose going on discovering remedies.

It is proposed now to consider the effects of the best and universally acknowledged specific remedies we possess in relationship to the above statements.

The simplest example to commence with is the action of iron in all forms in the type of anæmia known as chlorosis. Here we have to do with a specific remedy of such undoubted power that there are not more than two or three others such in the whole range of medicine. But does the knowledge of this specific remedy in the least degree diminish the incidence of chlorosis, or remove the plague from our midst? Not in the least; a very brief common-sense consideration of the problem shows that it cannot do so. An attack of chlorosis can be cut short in a given individual by treatment with iron salts, and if the individual changes her course of living, and goes on upon new hygienic conditions of diet and life and environment, the disease can be kept in most cases from recurring.

The specific remedy is good for the individual, but it has absolutely no effect upon the plague of the disease amongst the species. There will not be one case the less of chlorosis occurring for all the iron treatment in the world.

Chlorosis has considerably abated in recent years, but we have to search for the cause of this good result in other things than any treatment by a specific.

While chlorosis is sometimes seen in rapidly growing or neurotic girls of the better classes, it is essentially a disease of hard-worked, badly housed, and badly nourished girls and young women, of the working classes.

It is a disease of the domestic servant and shop-girl, and indoor female worker. To quote an eminent authority, Professor Osler: "The disease is most common among the ill-fed, overworked girls of large towns, who are confined all day in close, badly lighted rooms, or have to do much stair climbing." . . . "Lack of proper exercise and of fresh air, and the use of improper food, are important factors."

Now, how can any specific remedy, however beneficial to the individual, interfere with the vicious factors which produce chlorosis, followed by all the other fatal maladies, such as heart affections and tuberculosis, to which the enfeebled condition gives the inlet.

Not all the remedies of the most distinguished physician or most notorious nostrum-vendor can touch this problem. All the Blaud's pills ever manufactured, and the many millions of purgative Pink Pills for Pale People, might as well be poured down the sink, as far as stopping the attack of this disease on the young womanhood of the community is concerned.

This type of anæmia is abating because we are stopping the building of cellar and basement kitchens; the product of the days of snobs, when we could not live on the same floor as our maid-servants, and they had to run to underground burrows when we did not require their attentions. The lot of the shopgirl and workroom-girl has also improved. The State insists on workshops being ventilated and above-ground, and proper hours being kept. Still better things may be expected when "living-in" is made illegal. It takes no professional training to see which treatment is better for removing the disease chlorosis : treatment by drugs, or treatment by hygiene.

The iron treatment, combined with other things, is excellent for a chlorotic case; but there will not be one case less of chlorosis on account of it in a thousand years; on the other hand, improved conditions of living, working, and feeding have saved thousands from chlorosis, and will continue to do so still more as we become more civilised.

The next disease which we shall take as an example of this principle is one with which masses of the population of this country are riddled and destroyed in health and life itself. Like tuberculosis, it forms not one disease but many in its varying manifestations, and directly and indirectly, under many fanciful names, it kills nearly as many as tuberculosis. Like tuberculosis, it is an infectious disease, only possible of propagation because infected individuals by the tens of thousands exist in our midst, and no attempt whatever is made to isolate them or prevent them from transmitting the disease to others. Unlike the victims of phthisis, these diseased individuals know full well that they are passing on the contagion of this dread disease to their fellows; yet the community allows this criminality, this villainy, to go on without moving hand or foot to prevent it.

The most ghastly and fatal of our nervous diseases, including *locomotor ataxy* or *tabes dorsalis*, and *general paresis* or *general paralysis of the insane*, have now been shown to be due to the infective organism which is the only cause of this disease, that is blighting the lives of thousands of us.

Would to Heaven that the false sentimentality of the age could be thrown to the winds, and this loathsome disease attacked as it ought to be by the community! If we could only teach people that the Sin and the Crime consists not in speaking of this disease, but in concealing it and passing it on to those who are most innocent of all offence!

There is one way only in which we can save ourselves and our children and our children's children from this curse, and that is the same identical way in which we can rid ourselves of tuberculosis. They are both infectious diseases of chronic type, and there is one way, and but one, by which a civilised country can rid itself of them. In a single sentence, that way is, a National Medical Service, with compulsory powers of segregation of the unhealthy from the healthy.

In our present condition of education and civilisation one dare not, however, even mention the name of this disease in a book intended for general readers. So it shall be spoken of here by a name in fairly general use by medical men, viz., as "specific disease." The name suits the present purpose well, since it indicates that there is a "specific" treatment for this disease, which makes it *the* "specific disease" *par excellence.*

The medical profession has known for very many years two drugs which are specifics for this "specific disease" at different stages. Treatment by mercury or its compounds in the earlier stages is a definite cure nearly always successful when properly and adequately applied ; and similarly a substance called the iodide of potassium is specific in removing certain manifestations of the disease, which occur several years later in improperly treated cases. Here, then, if anywhere in all medicine, is a disease with its cure found out and well known.

If disease can be eradicated by finding out a cure for it, this disease ought to be eradicable. What are the facts? The disease is as widespread as ever, and shows no diminution. In out-patient or in-patient department of any of our hospitals, there are more patients with "specific disease" than with phthisis. Doctors in practice see and treat, by means of these specific cures, more cases of it than perhaps any other disease. They often cure it, too, as far as the individual who pays them is concerned; but meanwhile the brand has been passed along, and the disease laughs at all our puny efforts with "specifics." When are we going to be manly enough to attack it in the only way that can get rid of it?

The next instance which may be taken to illustrate the principle under discussion is one of the most glorious triumphs of modern scientific medicine, namely, Behring's discovery of the antitoxin of diphtheria.

Diphtheria kills in fatal cases by a most virulent poison, called a toxin, which the diphtheria germ produces where it grows in the throat, and this poison then is taken up into the blood and, passing round, poisons the heart and nervous system. The poison is most excessively deadly, as much so as snake venom, so that a small patch of diphtheritic growth in the throat can produce enough of this chemical poison to poison the whole body of the patient and cause death.

It is, strange to say, just this highly poisonous character that enables us to prepare the antidote, or antitoxin as it is called, because there is very little of the poison, and therefore it takes very little of the antidote to neutralise it. In other diseases there are formed much larger quantities of lower grade poisons, and we cannot prepare or administer sufficient amounts of the "anti" body to neutralise them. That is why we cannot extend the antitoxin cure for diphtheria to other infectious diseases; it has only been capable of extension to others, such as lockjaw, for example, where the disease poison is a very intense one, acting in minute quantities.

The diphtheria antidote, or antitoxin, is made by choosing out a more resistant animal against diphtheria, such as the horse, and injecting into this animal the dead bodies of the diphtheria organism containing plenty of the diphtheria poison. This sets up a chemical reaction in the horse's body, in which the antidote is manufactured to neutralise the poison. Some *excess* of the antidote is made by the horse's body during this process, and this excess is present in the fluid part of the horse's blood. On now drawing off some of the horse's blood, which can be done almost painlessly by opening a vein in the neck, the horse going on quietly eating all the time, and by separating afterwards the fluid part of the horse's blood, the specific remedy for diphtheria is obtained, called "diphtheria antitoxin."

So much by way of prefatory explanation; the next point is that, by general accord of the medical profession throughout the whole world, it is agreed that this treatment is most efficient, and indeed specific for diphtheria. The mortality rate of cases properly treated with antitoxin at an early stage is enormously less than that of untreated cases.

In fact, we have a specific cure here by an organic or bio-chemical drug, as great as the two we have just discussed previously. Anything which follows is meant as no disparagement of this brilliant discovery, but merely by admitting the intrinsic value of diphtheria antitoxin, applied properly in sufficient amount at the right time as a specific cure for each case of diphtheria, to drive home *à fortiori* that a disease cannot be eradicated by means of a cure, but will continue to be a plague to the community, and will still go on destroying valuable lives, until a proper system of dealing with it is devised.

In cases occurring in well-to-do families, almost as soon as the child is ill the doctor is sent for, and diphtheria being diagnosed, the antitoxic treatment is at once efficiently applied without waiting to take any chances as to whether the case is going to be a mild or a serious one. The consequence is an enormous decrease in the diphtheria death-rate in this class of practice. Diphtheria antitoxin is the sheet-anchor of the practitioner attending to the middle classes, and he recognises and owns it everywhere.

But contrast this with what happens in the case of the poor. Here the child is allowed to go about with its sore throat and illness for two or three days; the mother may be out all day at work, or, failing this, may have all the work at home to do for her own large family, husband, and probably lodgers; all the cooking, washing, and cleaning to do for the entire household. Little wonder that each child cannot receive as much care and attention as in a middle-class family. One of the children goes about with a sore throat, supposed to be an ordinary sore throat of a rather bad type. This throat is treated with domestic remedies and according to the advice of all and sundry of the neighbour women, who come with their children in arms, and at their knee, to look at this mysterious sore throat and, incidentally, get their children infected.

Probably for a day or two the child goes to school with "only a sore throat," giving rise to a crop of bad sore throats in the neighbourhood. Finally the poison of the diphtheria germ, circulating in the blood, makes the child so ill that at last a doctor is sent for, who diagnoses diphtheria, and may at once give "antitoxin" (it is necessarily a very expensive substance, from its mode of preparation), or may notify the case and have it removed to a municipal infectious disease hospital, when at last it gets its first dose of antitoxin.[1] It is obvious

---

[1] No antitoxin is allowed in most Poor Law Infirmaries, to the many cases of diphtheria treated there. See Poor Law Commission Report.

I

that the poison has a long start of the antidote, and it is little wonder, since the large
majority of cases of diphtheria in the country
are treated in this latter way, that the death-
rate from diphtheria has only slightly decreased since the introduction of the antitoxin
treatment.

Our present system of administration and
treatment of infectious diseases amongst the
working classes is responsible for this more
than partial failure to adequately decrease the
death-rate from diphtheria.

The facts of the diphtheria death-rate furnish
the proof for the second proposition stated
above, viz. that "the possession of a most
powerful specific remedy for a given disease,
*with our present-day modes of practice and
employing it,* may produce little or no effect
upon the death-rate from the disease."

Here, at five-year intervals, are the total
numbers of deaths from diphtheria (excluding
croup) recorded annually in each year mentioned in the United Kingdom. It may be
mentioned that in the earlier years a certain
number of cases of diphtheria were probably
recorded as "croup" on account of less perfect means of diagnosis, but this does not
so materially vitiate the comparison as to
destroy the proof of the principle mentioned
above.

TOTAL ANNUAL DEATHS FROM DIPHTHERIA IN
UNITED KINGDOM

Year						Deaths
1881	.	.	.	.	.	4,292
1886	.	.	.	.	.	5,017
1891	.	.	.	.	.	6,147
1896	.	.	.	.	.	9,987
1901	.	.	.	.	.	10,013
1906	.	.	.	.	.	7,258

So much for the death-rate; now as to the
incidence of the disease, which is the important criterion on our scientific methods, and
that which matters as far as the health of the
race is concerned. Here, so far as statistics
can be found, there is no diminution whatever.
Nor, if we will only look at the problem in a
philosophical and logical way, can there be
any reasonable expectation of any decrease.
Granting that a specific remedy can cut short
an attack and save an individual patient, and
that so, when we learn to apply our remedy
all round, and at the proper time, and in the
proper way, the death-rate may and must fall;
yet this has nothing to do with the incidence
of fresh cases unless the specific remedy cuts
out the disease before it is infectious, and that
is a very long cry from where we stand. During
the days when the diphtheritic child is going
to school; when it is being doctored by the
mother in the midst of its brothers and sisters,
in a two or three room tenement, and sleeping
with some of them in the same bed at night;

when it is being visited and prescribed for by the
neighbour wives accompanied by their children,
who try to see into its throat at the same time
as the mothers; during all this time where does
the specific remedy come into the problem?

Until our united wisdom discovers some way
of removing children suffering from diphtheria
to isolation conditions *at once* without waiting
till the case is brought in the present orthodox
way under the notice of the doctor, *children are
going to continue dying of diphtheria by the
thousand*. When we do find out how to do
our work, then Behring's discovery will help us
to cure the individual case from slum as at present in villa, and more rapidly to eradicate the
disease; till then, the big death-roll continues.

The most illustrative case of all is that with
which we shall conclude our examination of
medication versus hygiene in the warfare with
disease. The subject is almost as fascinating
as a romance in its entrancing interest; it is
the story of the combat of modern science with
malaria.

Fortunately for the inhabitants of the United
Kingdom, our well-drained soil and climatic
conditions at present preserve us free from the
ague or malaria; although in earlier days it was
common enough in the Fen Country. In other
regions of the earth, over extensive areas, it
attacks millions of people and does enormous
damage, not only by the great death-roll directly
due to the disease itself, but by the lowering of

vitality induced by repeated attacks so producing continually ill-health and diminished resistance to other diseases. In ancient days malaria was one of the most prominent diseases amidst the Romans, and probably did much to sap the vigour and physique of that dominant race towards its decline. Malaria is still the scourge of modern Italy; hundreds of thousands of the inhabitants of the United States of America are afflicted by it; it has earned for West Africa the appellation of "the white man's grave"; and thousands of the natives of India die annually directly from its ravages.

Yet this is the disease to which we have known a specific, in quinine, for the past two hundred and seventy years.

A South American Indian used Cinchona, or Jesuits' bark, to cure a Jesuit missionary prostrated by fever. The same bark was used as a cure for the Countess of Cinchon in 1638. Afterwards the Jesuit brotherhood disseminated a knowledge of its virtues throughout Europe.

Long researches, into the details of which we cannot here enter, laid bare the fact that this activity of the bark was due to a substance contained in it called *quinine*. This substance forms beautiful white salts with certain acids, and nowadays these salts are isolated in large quantities and used medicinally in this country, and exported abroad to malaria-ridden countries such as India and West and Central Africa. Small amounts of this active principle, quinine, can be made to take the place of very much greater quantities of bark extract, and in the form of powder and tablets, quinine is an essential in all expeditions for exploration, settlement, or sport undertaken by white men in the tropics, and in all tropical and sub-tropical colonies or stations inhabited by white men.

For most ordinary attacks of malaria, quinine is an absolute specific; but with prolonged exposure to infection and recurrent attacks it loses its power, and there are some cases especially resistant to it. It may, however, be placed amongst the four or five *true specifics* known to medicine.

All this progress and discovery of the specific remedy had been realised purely empirically, without any real experimental knowledge having been obtained, apart from theorising, as to how malaria was caused. We shall now trace out in brief outline how the cause of malaria was discovered; how man was shown to become infected by a peculiar and interesting agent, and how this discovery, by showing the rational way to avoid infection, has almost banished malaria from districts where it was a veritable scourge.

The name of the disease, malaria, shows that it was early associated in men's minds with bad air; for centuries it was believed to be due to " miasmata " or stagnant vapours arising from the marshes. But it has remained for the scientific work of the experimental medicine

of the immediate past generation to clear up
this riddle of the ages as to the true origin and
nature of malarial fever.

The most remarkable symptom of the disease
which puzzled the physicians for centuries,
namely, the ordered sequence of events in each
attack, first became capable of being understood
when the scientific work had laid bare the true
causation of the disease.

The characteristic symptom of malarial fever
is the onset at regular intervals of time of acute
attacks, each with a rhythmic sequence of events,
at regular periods. Between these attacks the
patient is fairly well, though somewhat exhausted.

In each attack there is a cold stage, a hot
stage, and then a stage of excessive perspiration followed by relief from pain and other
symptoms. There is no real drop in body
temperature when the patient is complaining
of cold, but rather a rise, yet the patient feels
intensely cold ; the teeth chatter, and he shivers
at intervals most violently ; the skin is shrivelled
and the face and hands blue ; there are agonising pains in the back and limbs.

After a variable period up to three hours, this
phase is succeeded rapidly by the hot stage,
in which the face becomes flushed, but as yet
there is no perspiration ; there is racking head-
ache, and sometimes delirium, and the patient
feels restless and burning hot all over. This
agonising stage lasts from one to four or five

hours, when a blessed relief comes with the sweating stage, in which the patient loses the severe pain and becomes tired and sleepy, temperature falls, and pulse and respiration slack off as the attack dies down.

The explanation of this sequence was given when Laveran, a French observer, discovered that malaria was due to a minute organism existing in the blood and undergoing a life-cycle of changes corresponding in its time period to these rhythmic onsets of fever.

Each generation of this blood parasite discovered by Laveran bursts out, or spores, at a certain time, and this it is which causes the malarial attack. The next malarial attack occurs when the next sporing or swarming occurs, again discharging poison into the blood.

The blood normally contains, suspended in its fluid, immense numbers of little bodies called *red blood corpuscles*, and it is in these blood corpuscles that Laveran's parasites live and grow. At a certain stage they break the corpuscles up simultaneously, so destroying a certain percentage of the patient's blood, and also carrying out poisonous substances into the circulation. Then there is an attack. At the same time the living parasitic spores so set free begin to enter fresh corpuscles of the blood, and start a new cycle, the consummation of which is a fresh outbreak and a fresh attack, and so the cycle continues to be repeated.

The remainder of the problem, although strongly reminiscent of King George the Third and a simple problem of cookery connected with apple dumplings, defeated the best efforts of scientists for many years. With its solution came the first practical victories in the warfare with malaria. The still unsolved part of the puzzle was how the malarial parasite of Laveran got into the blood-corpuscles, and what was the connection with the marshes.

Two British observers have shared the honour of supplying this portion of the history in quite recent years, the original suggestion being made by Sir Patrick Manson, and the patient and brilliant work of Ronald Ross supplying the accurate proof. The most carefully elaborated work of Ross demonstrated that the above-mentioned sporulating cycle occurring in human blood did not form the complete life-cycle of the parasite, but had to be refreshed and supplemented after a certain number of generations, by a sexual cycle, according to a very well-known law for many lowly animal organisms.

This second cycle was shown by Ross to occur in the stomachs of certain species of mosquitoes of a particular genus called *Anopheles*, which breeds in the marshes and small ponds and puddles near malaria-ridden districts. Many species of mosquito are quite harmless, being unsuitable for this refreshing of the strain of parasite, but a particular species of mosquito of this genus *Anopheles* was examined at different periods, after feeding on malarial blood, by Ross, and the mosquito was found to develop this special cycle of the malarial parasite in glands of the stomach.

It was shown that a mosquito of the right species, a certain time after biting a patient, became infective, and was capable now of carrying malaria to another human being, but only after the parasite had undergone the necessary metamorphoses in the mosquito's stomach.

The minute and careful work necessary to show such changes going on in the glands of a structure so delicate as the stomach of a mosquito, can be appreciated. Another point of view of great beauty is the exquisite bio-chemical adaptation in Nature which requires one particular breed of mosquito in order to provide just the proper chemical nutrition for the induction of this particular cycle of life in the malarial parasite, a cycle most essentially different from the cycle occurring in human blood, and giving rise to the patient's attacks.

The exquisite beauty of this adaptation, from the bio-chemist's point of view, will be appreciated when it is stated that the, as yet unknown but quite certainly existent, organism of yellow-fever is borne by a different kind or genus of mosquito known as *Stegomyia.*

Let us turn now to what intimately concerns us here, namely, the application of the reflected light of the successes in this problem of attack upon malaria to the attack on the consumption problem in our own country.

The initial intention in quoting malaria was to show that here, where for generations one of the best, if not indeed the most notable, specifics of all medicine, had existed and been universally applied, the disease had still gone on rampantly ravaging, without abatement, the populaces of the countries. Quinine had been of very great and undeniable advantage *to the individual,* but of little or none *to the race.*

Let us now carry our account of malaria one step farther and see how we can reap a great lesson for application to the huge problem of tuberculosis.

It is clear, even from the short outline given above, that *the only way,* under natural conditions, in which a new individual in a malarial country can be stricken by malaria, is by being bitten by the right species of mosquito, viz. by the *Anopheles.* This is confirmed by the well-substantiated discovery that, marshes or no marshes, where there are no *Anopheles* mosquitoes there is no malaria. The logical outcome is that if we can prevent people being bitten by these mosquitoes in any way—either by protecting, by mosquito netting, etc., from the insects, or, preferably, and more perfectly, by ridding the district of the disease-bearing *Anopheles*—then we simply cut off malaria.

Let us carry in our minds here the corresponding parallel for tuberculosis; here, there

is no intermediate thing in the way of a mosquito, but it is just as true that *no person in this
World gets consumption otherwise than from
another consumptive*, and if we segregate off
consumptives by themselves, in many ways an
easier problem and less expensive than removing
mosquitoes from a district of country, we shall
undoubtedly reap all those advantages which
are about to be described in relationship to
malaria, and in a surprisingly short period tuberculosis will be almost unknown.

Space forbids entering into the details of the
several successful campaigns against malaria by
mosquito destruction, the only rational method ;
but it may be stated that in no instance where
the somewhat difficult problems of thorough
drainage have been solved, or removal of dwell-
ings from the vicinity of mosquito-rearing
swamps has been effected, has there failed of
reaping the due reward in decrease of malaria
and death from malarial fever; and, in some
instances, districts which were previously decimated, such as Ismailia in Egypt, and Conakry
on the West Coast of Africa, are now almost
free from the scourge.

The problem of practical sanitation is made
somewhat lighter by the fact that the parasite-
bearing mosquitoes do not fly far from the
shallow pools in which they deposit their eggs,
so that they may be swarming in a particular
spot, and another district, a few hundred yards
or a quarter of a mile away, may be quite free

from them. A second factor of assistance is
that the larvæ, in order to develop farther, must
at a certain stage reach the air at the surface of
the water, and hence by sprinkling petroleum
or creosote over the pools and marshes their
development may be prevented.

The hygienic measures indicated in fighting
malaria are accordingly drainage and filling up
of pools around houses, looking after cisterns
and other water surfaces, and disinfection of
surfaces of water by oil where removal is impossible, within, say, a radius of one mile around
a given town or community which it is desired
to protect.

Some towns and situations are more ideally
placed for such treatment than others, and in
certain test cases, where communities were
decimated by malaria, and where surface conditions and isolation lent themselves to treatment by the above methods, the disease has
been practically stamped out. It may be added,
as a particularly interesting example, that in
Central America the main obstacle to completion of the great undertaking of the Panama
Canal was the health of the workmen, and
that now malaria and yellow-fever (which, as
mentioned above, is also a mosquito-borne disease) have been almost crushed out in this
district by the American Medical Service, the
work is being pushed forward to completion
under healthy conditions. When this great
Panama Canal is at length opened, it will be

a united triumph for both Engineering and Medical Science.

The methods to conquer tuberculosis must be conceived on somewhat different lines; each disease has its own problems of detail, but essentially the rationale must be the same. When we know how a disease is spread, and that it possesses no other method of attack unknown to us, then we must throw all the strength of our Medical Service and the knowledge of our science into stopping the means of spread, instead of supinely contenting ourselves with tinkering the individual. Incidentally, however, the actual victim of attack is given a better chance than ever before when our scheme is laid on these new scientific lines.

Returning now to the summing up of our main proposition regarding specific cures for disease, we have *demonstrated* by taking the four best established specific cures in all medicine—viz. (1) iron in anæmia, (2) mercury in "specific disease," (3) antitoxin in diphtheria, and (4) quinine in malaria—that in none of these cases is the race relieved from suffering and death by the existence of a cure for the individual.

The fact, now we have found it, and proved it, and tested it, is worth reiterating and dinning into the ears of the World, so that it may awake from drugging itself to sleep and death.

There is only one way given under Heaven

by which disease can be abolished, and a finer
and fitter race evolved, and that is by stopping
the causes of disease, and throwing all our force
into the resistance of its spread. If we are
brave enough to do this, we shall, it is true,
save millions of money every year, but we shall
also achieve something nobler and grander than
this which cannot be stamped upon coins of
gold or written down on cheques or bank-notes.

Coming now to the details of a rational
national attack upon the disease, tuberculosis,
we may first of all sketch what is at present
being done in the way of attack. We possess
certain hospitals provided by the charitable for
consumption, and certain sanatoria in healthy
districts, both for those who can pay and also
for a few of those who cannot. What are these
institutions doing to-day for the consumptive
patient and for the community; are our efforts
anything like commensurate, or are we merely
wasting time and money on a little child's
play?

The orthodox position taken up by the
medical profession and by Medical Officers of
Health in regard to the danger of infection by
tuberculosis, is well illustrated by the following
extracts from the Annual Report of the Medical
Officer of Health of a great English city.

These extracts are quoted here, not in order
to criticise any one person's views, but because
they so clearly represent a widespread doctrine

which it is thought desirable to examine carefully in the public interest.

"The susceptibility of the individual who inhales or swallows the bacilli varies ; constitutional predisposition, the habits, the occupation, the intemperance of the exposed person may prepare the way for it. In numberless cases the likelihood is that the bacillus is swallowed or inhaled without any ill effect."

"It will be seen, therefore, that the consumptive patient must not be always and under all circumstances regarded as a source of danger to others."

"Forms of tuberculosis other than phthisis may be regarded as practically non-infectious."[1] "The large majority of the cases of phthisis come under the same category, whilst the remainder are infectious only under circumstances favourable to infection, and have little, if any, tendency to spread where reasonable precautions can be adopted."

It may be remarked that elsewhere it is stated in the same report that "A careless patient in bad surroundings may easily become a source of infection."

The very danger of some of these statements lies in the fact that they are true, such as that "the consumptive patient must not be always and under all circumstances regarded as a source of danger to others." This is perfectly true,

[1] This statement standing alone may be accepted ; it is quoted in order to be able to properly quote the context.

but stated in this way and brought to the attention of laymen, it may easily induce a false sense of security which may be of great danger. It may readily induce slackness of action in removing cases of danger, if the danger is taken so lightly. Any patient producing sputum containing tubercular germs and living at large in the community is a very great source of danger indeed, and amongst the poorer classes probably three cases out of four possess this criterion of danger. If we except a *possible* small percentage of infection carried in milk, all infection comes directly from other tubercular patients. After all, we *are* dealing with an infectious disease, even if it be a chronic one. If we could only see the patients hit by the infection in phthisis as we do in smallpox, the present order of things would not long be tolerated. There is no possible doubt that they are hit just as much as they would be by smallpox, but phthisis is insidious in its onset, and so we blink at the cause and do not remove it.

The statement that "In numberless cases the likelihood is that the bacillus is swallowed or inhaled without any ill effect" crystallises a common doctrine that all the time we are swallowing various deadly germs which do us no harm because we have a strong resistance, or *immunity*, as it is called. This is carrying the immunity doctrine to an entirely unwarrantable extent. There exists no clear evidence regarding immunity, either natural or

K

acquired, in the case of phthisis. All the experimental evidence of the bacteriological laboratory lies in the opposite direction. It appears to be true of phthisis, as of pneumonia, that, instead of protecting, one attack, if anything, predisposes to another. At any rate, there is much evidence accumulating that numbers of sanatorium cures which apparently relapse are truly re-infections with the disease.

The evidence from thousands of autopsies has shown the existence of old healed tubercular injuries in the bodies of people dying from other diseases. This shows that we all possess powers of resistance against tuberculosis, and that many people, if not all, are capable of infection with the disease; but there is no clear evidence that some individuals possess enormous resistance and others very feeble powers of resistance. Repeated deaths in the same family do not prove this; they only prove closer proximity, and hence more efficient and repeated infection. The Appendix at the end of the book on relative death-rates in different occupations proves this clearly; for example, *one* printer in every *three* dies of phthisis, but only *one* clergyman in every *twenty-six* dies of it. Surely, such figures can only mean that the printer in his occupation runs, for some reason, about nine times as much chance of infection as the clergyman in his, and not that the clergyman's body possesses naturally ninefold the immunity of the printer's body.

In any case, whatever we may believe regarding immunity, this point is aside from the main issue, which is that there is such a great number of us open to infection by our fellows, and, under present wrong conditions, so often subjected to infection, that seventy-five thousand of us die every year.   It matters not to the argument that ten times as many may be infected each year and recover on account of better resistance ; both those who die, and those who escape from the jaws of death, were infected by other sufferers, and by inhaling or swallowing tubercle bacilli.

No one of any scientific authority has ever claimed that tubercle bacilli are to be found in mouth or sputum except in the case of individuals suffering from tuberculosis.   On what possible scientific ground, then, can the opinion be based that the tubercle bacillus can be swallowed or inhaled without any ill effect ?

There is no such scientific ground, and the present writer ventures to make the counter statement that *in over seventy thousand cases every year in this country alone people* DIE *because they have swallowed or inhaled living tubercle bacilli, produced and cultured in the lungs of consumptive patients living or working near them.* The further statement may be added that each of these seventy thousand people induces the disease in one other person before he dies, and that in this way a new seventy thousand people are prepared for next year's sacrifice to this disease.

These are facts that the inhabitants of the country have to deal with, and not fancies. There is no doubt that in the earlier stages the consumptive is not so dangerous as later, and also that the educated consumptive is less dangerous than the ignorant consumptive; but the dreadful average is that, one with another, each consumptive starts a new victim on the road to death before he himself departs.   The statement has all the crushing force of a mathematical demonstration : how otherwise is the disease kept up ?   Is it done by the milk of a small number of tuberculous cows ?   Why, then, not have them slaughtered at once ?   Every tubercular animal in the country ought, of course, to be slaughtered at once, and perchance with more energy and inspection we could find annually a few more than we do now; but, surely, we do not believe that any serious percentage of phthisis is carried in this way.   The only remaining way is from one human being to another.

One final criticism of the statement that the *large majority* of the cases of phthisis are practically non-infectious, whilst the remainder are infectious only under circumstances favourable to infection, and have little if any tendency to spread where reasonable precautions can be adopted.   The accuracy of this may be questioned ; but, if true, surely the logical reply is, why not isolate the *small minority* which are infectious under unfavourable circumstances, or adopt such reasonable precautions that the disease loses its tendency to spread?

These statements need not have detained us so long were it not that they reflect the current orthodox view of many people keenly interested in this great problem and truly anxious for its solution.

One can also recognise and honour the kindly spirit which, on account of the attitude of the public towards the consumptive patient, tends to allay the growing feeling that it is unsafe to work or associate closely with the sufferers from this disease.

Still, with all desire to make the lot of the consumptive a happier one and his life easier, objects which can be attained in other and safer ways, we must be most careful that we look also at the side of the case of the healthy members of the community, and safeguard them from death, and their families from destitution.

It is necessary here that we should not let a weak sentimentality run away with us, and this public distrust of the consumptive is a most salutary public feeling. There is no doubt whatever that an operative or worker, in nearly all workshops and indoor occupations, who is at that stage of the disease that he is producing sputum is a real danger, and a great danger, to other workers all around him. To the personal knowledge of the writer, there are hundreds of such consumptive workers in textile works, many of them weavers who suck the shuttles in threading them, these shuttles being later redistributed and reaching other workers, and the danger of employment of these workers to other workers in the same shop is enormous.

Until some national scheme is devised, let workers subscribe funds to send their consumptive co-workers to sanatoria, and let them demand a certificate of freedom from infectivity before such workers are re-admitted to work in the shop. But it is pure folly and madness to keep on working beside them, and the Board of Trade ought to see that it is stopped.

Workpeople ought to strike against present conditions, both on account of the sick people and on their own account. Present conditions consign the sick to a living death, and the healthy to be ready to step into the ranks of death in turn.

The view that the germs of consumption are being swallowed daily by all of us in the dust from our roads without injury or infection, on account of our great virility and powers of resistance, while most comforting to the strong, is probably, indeed almost certainly, a pure myth. If it were so, that we so swallowed and inhaled live tuberculosis germs, the population of the earth would have rapidly dwindled, especially since the advent of the motor-car; but there is no shred or tatter of scientific evidence for this view. The most expert bacteriologist would frequently fail to obtain live tuberculosis germs from blown road dust. It would be a very bad day for us all if they were present. The tubercular infection is usually carried round from man to man much fresher than this, and while it is all-important, so long as thousands of dangerous sputum-producing consumptives are allowed free in our midst, that they should be taught not to spit, do let us remember that this regulation alone is but playing at things, and that there are a hundred and one ways in which the phthisical patient passes on the living germs, many of them much more dangerous than spitting.

Fortunately for us, the bacillus of tuberculosis is an exceedingly delicate organism, of which the vitality is more readily destroyed than that of most of the micro-organisms of disease. In the laboratory it can only be grown upon special culture media, refusing to grow on ordinary nutrients upon which most of our ordinary disease-producing microbes flourish. It is very delicate and slow in its growth, and perishes readily under variations of external conditions. Sunlight destroys it rapidly, like most other bacteria, and it is nearly always killed by complete drying. It is hence exceedingly probable that a great deal of consumption is borne by *moist* sputum, or by sputum not long exposed to air and light, from patient to patient. It is those brought very close to the consumptive, and living the same

life as the consumptive, inhabiting the same
small rooms, sleeping in the same bed, using
the same vessels for eating or drinking, handling
the same articles and the same tools, who are
most liable to infection.

The evidence as to non-infection of physicians
and nurses in chest hospitals does not run
counter to this at all. Patients live an entirely
different life at hospital as to sanitary régime,
reception of sputum in special vessels into
antiseptics, washing of the hands, etc. Again,
the nurses and doctors handle but little
that is previously handled by the patients,
eating utensils are thoroughly cleansed, and
the same things are not used by nurses and
patients. The whole life is different from the
patient's home-life, and the relations to him
of doctor and nurse are essentially different
from the relations of his relatives, friends, and
co-workers. Such evidence is worth nothing;
one might as well claim, because doctors and
nurses do not contract typhoid fever from a
patient, that in the good old days, when we
treated typhoid as we now treat consumption,
a typhoid patient could not infect persons in
his neighbourhood; and tubercular infection,
from what we know as to the two channels
of infection, is obviously more easily distributed
than typhoid, which can only come from fæcal
contamination.

The lay public probably but feebly realises
how little is done at present by either Public

Health Authorities or Hospital Authorities to stop the spread of consumption, and how little powers they possess to enable them to stop the dangerous consumptive from going forth unhealed to lay death-traps for the rest of the community.

It is well that the matter should be set forth in black and white before the general public, and our public bodies and legislators, so that there may no longer be the excuse that "We did not know that these things were so."

It may be stated at the outset, to prevent any misunderstanding, that no blame attaches to any particular person or any institution here given as an example or a concrete case; the things portrayed below are done everywhere throughout the length and breadth of the land, and there is no legislation and no organisation to prevent their being done.

Let us commence with a personal experience of a concrete case, the patient coming from one of the best and most scientifically conducted Consumptive Hospitals in the Kingdom—an institution with a fine laboratory, efficient staff, and all clinical facilities; but what avail all these good things if the patient himself is to be sole arbiter and judge of when he is to leave hospital and cast himself forth free again into the great sea of humanity?

The case related simply came under the author's notice from this institution, and the study of that case first awakened his mind, and allowed him to perceive how we are everywhere working at present, and how futile all our labours must be until we work differently. Otherwise this case was just like thousands of others elsewhere and everywhere.

About two years ago, certain results obtained in the laboratory on exposing growths of the bacillus of tuberculosis to increased percentages of oxygen gas, whereby the germs are killed, suggested the experiment of causing tubercular patients to breathe oxygen for a considerable period daily.

By the courtesy of the Staff of the hospital, the author was placed in communication with a patient who came to the laboratory and breathed oxygen for an hour daily. The patient's sputum was examined regularly for the tubercle bacillus at intervals during the whole period of about six months: the result of the examination varied—sometimes bacilli were present, and sometimes they were absent. Between two and three months after the commencement of the experiment, the patient, who did not appear to be getting worse in general health, but rather better, expressed his intention of leaving the hospital *to look for employment*, but said that he was willing to continue the oxygen inhalations at the laboratory until he found employment. At this time his sputum contained tubercle bacilli.

Now, here is the position: a patient whose

sputum contains the germs of a deadly infectious disease declares that he wishes to leave hospital and return to the community and to work, and the hospital authorities have neither the power by legislation, nor the accommodation in the way of beds, to prevent him. At the moment at which this patient wants to leave, he belongs to that great category of consumptive hospital patients who are returned on the hospital books as leaving the institution "improved in health." There is no time to wait for any completeness of recovery in either hospital or sanatorium, for there are plenty more patients, forming most prolific tuberculosis-germ factories, distributed out amongst the public and waiting their turn for admission to the hospitals.

Returning now to our particular patient, the author, being most anxious to finish his experiment, subsidised this patient for a period of over three months, during which time he came daily to the laboratory. During this period he was producing tuberculosis germs all the time, living with his people at home, and going about daily looking for employment, just as were hundreds more in the city like him.

How under our present system could he be doing otherwise? He was a skilled workman almost out of benefit in his club, and without other means to support himself and his wife, who took in laundry work. A little money came occasionally from a son, a ship's steward in irregular employment, who, by the bye, lived

at home when off his ship or out of work.
Can the reader begin to catch any glimmering
of appreciation of how we propagate tuberculosis by our present system?

This particular patient was a person of most
cleanly habits of person and conduct, most
amenable to good advice for the protection of
himself and others, as "harmless a consumptive," within the meaning of the phrase, as
could well be imagined, and who had had his
hospital drill. He never expectorated in a
wrongful way, even once, in the whole period.
His habits were made the subject of careful
watching by the writer during the experiment.
He had the rapidly repeated cough of the
consumptive, and nearly always put his hand
before his mouth when he coughed; sometimes,
as with every one, little particles of moisture
were produced in coughing, and there is no
doubt that these often reached the hand and
infected it. He also frequently rubbed his lips
and moustache with his hand quite uncon-
sciously. It was quite obvious that both mouth
and hands of this patient could convey infection
to any one using the same things as he had
touched with mouth or hands.

The reader can readily construct for himself,
by reflecting upon the many ways we come in
contact, directly or indirectly, with our fellow-
men, or they come in contact with _our_ food or
clothing or persons, how many chances there
are, if they are infected with tuberculosis, for

the infection being carried fresh and moist to
us. There is, the reader may be assured, no
need to invoke dried sputum blown up with
road dust. Any one who for a day or two will
just take observations, and reflect upon them,
can prove the matter for himself, that the more
consumptives there are about unrestrained, the
more chance of infection there is for himself
and all other healthy people.

Let us take a few examples to illustrate the
matter, not with the object of making our daily
lives a terror, but of stirring up some sane spirit
of objection to things as they are, and developing strength of public opinion, which may put
an end to the present régime.

Suppose we take a journey by tramcar or
train : the conductor or ticket clerk who punches
our ticket may in the present condition of the
law be a sputum-producing consumptive—a fair
number of tram-conductors die of the disease
every year ;[1] probably just before he punched
your ticket he had his fingers in his mouth, or
applied them to stop a cough. Having held
your ticket in your hand, you probably soon
after may touch your own mouth with your
fingers—most people do at times; it is a
habit acquired in early infancy, and some of
us never lose it.

Suppose next you require some wearing ap-

[1] *One* tramway conductor, out of every *four* dying, dies of
consumption. See Appendix at end of the volume, third
occupation given in table, p. 201.

parel, such as a new suit of clothes. You go to
a most respectable shop; but the tailor sends
the work nearly always to some sweating den
in the slums, in the Jewish quarter of the city
most probably, where tuberculosis is often most
particularly rampant.[1]   Have you ever watched
a sweated foreign tailor at work ? If you had, you
would agree that if he were tubercular, and had
tubercle bacilli in his sputum, both his hands
and his work would soon be infected.   This
work comes home to you, respectably and neatly
done up, and you suspect no danger.   But, on
the whole, now you think of it, would it not be
to the public interest if all tubercular tailors
were sent to healthy sanatoria; would it not be
better both for tailors and for you ?

Let us now wade a little deeper into the
matter and consider how food supplies are
handled.   Fortunately for our peace of mind,
most of what happens to them is hidden from
our eyes.   Still, it is better for the problem we
are dealing with not to hide our noses in the
sands, so let us, for once in a way, just look at
that small part of the process more easily visible
to us.

Last night the writer went into a shop and
bought half a pound of biscuits, and watched
them being put up.   Each biscuit was touched
by the grocer's hand as it was put in the bag.
One biscuit fell on the floor; it was promptly

---

[1] In the tailoring trade, about one in six dies of consumption.

lifted up and put on the counter; its fate after the customer left the shop remains unknown to him. Now suppose that grocer were ill of phthisis—many grocers die of phthisis every year[1]—and just finish painting the picture for yourself.

If you will watch your greengrocer as he handles strawberries and other fruit which you afterwards eat fresh without any cooking or other process of sterilisation—and soon, too, after he has handled it—you will also agree that a tubercular greengrocer may be a source of infection for others.[2]

Returning again to a little touch of personal experience, recently, when going upon a picnic in the country, an emergency supply of extra milk was required. A visit to a local dairy procured a supply, and standing at the doorway, one distinctly observed the dairymaid put her forefinger into the pan of milk and stir it around, to mix up cream and milk, before measuring out the supply. One's first impulse was to refuse the milk, but after all it was an accident that the incident had been observed. Given that the dairymaid was healthy and her forefinger clean, it did not matter so much. But milk is an excellent culture medium for germs, and often contains more than the innocent cow is responsible for.

---

[1] One grocer out of every eight dies of this disease.
[2] The consumption death-rate for fruiterers and green-grocers is one in eight.

About six years ago, the author noticed that a milk-carrier, who also milked the cows at the dairy where he was employed and then took round the milk in a first-class district, was phthisical. Being interested in the case, he talked with the man on his return after a certain period of absence, and found he had been a patient in hospital during the interval. For months this man was observed carrying round the milk, dispensing it at the doors, and growing gradually weaker and weaker with phthisis. This consumptive carried the milk round a large district until he grew so weak that he could carry it no longer, and a few weeks later he died in hospital *of phthisis*.

There is no law, not even any well-defined public feeling, to prevent this sort of thing; but is it right?

Consider next our public habits of eating and drinking. Men suffer more from tuberculosis than women, and the death-rate amongst women is dropping far more rapidly than the male death-rate. There is little doubt that this difference is due to differences in habits. Women spend their day (apart from female public-works employments) more in the home; they eat and drink, and come in contact with things outside the family circle, far less than men. Workmen in public workshops drink water or beer or other fluids often from the same public drinking cups and vessels. If there is a workman with active phthisis amongst them, every time he uses the common drinking vessel he probably sets a death-trap for the man who comes next after him, for the cup is not carefully cleansed on its rim after each draught. If any one doubts the possibility of such contagion, let him perform this experiment. Take a drink from a glass of milk and set it down on the table; look then at the place where your lips have touched it on the rim, inside and outside. Suppose now that a workman in a crowded shop had left a drinking cup like that, he being a consumptive, and now, without the cup being washed, another man came after him and drank, using the same part of the cup rim, would the second comer run no chance of infection?

It is interesting, to any one who may have the opportunity, to watch how the drinking of beer is carried on at the workman's side of the British Public House. Often a quart of beer is consumed by four workmen from the same pewter pot, the men drinking in turn. A beautiful, sentimental, loving-cup arrangement, the four jolly chums drinking in a community of good fellowship. Suppose one of the four to have phthisis, as is often the case, then the cup may well be a cup of death. Even when drinking in common is not resorted to, the methods for rinsing—one can scarce call it cleansing—the pewter pots and glasses are of the most meagre description. They are usually passed through a sink and wiped by

L

a cloth which has previously wiped many dozen others.

Perhaps enough has been said to show how seventy-five thousand new consumptives are enlisted into this big battalion of disease every year, and we may now turn to the more cheerful subject of reform, and the stoppage of this enlistment.

A complete scheme for the entire United Kingdom for the eradication of tuberculosis would cost between seven and eight million pounds annually for a period of five years, after which the cost of maintaining the disease in abeyance would not exceed one million pounds annually. As tuberculosis now costs at least ten millions annually in direct expenditure, and another twenty millions annually in indirect expenditure, the new scheme would mean a considerable saving even during the first five years; but, of course, the cost of it would have to come from imperial taxation instead of, as at present, partially from private pockets and partially from municipal and Poor Law boards.

In addition to the annual expenditure in maintenance of the scheme for five or six years during the period of eradication, there would be required a capital sum of ten millions at the outset for the provision of sanatoria for the occupation of the 100,000 actively infectious cases of tuberculosis, which, as we shall see presently, is about the number for which we should have to make provision.

This sum allows an average amount of £100 for the provision of each bed, and as the sanatoria need only be temporary buildings, such a sum would be quite adequate.

As this initial cost of £10,000,000 is required to stamp out what is an enormous annual drain on the nation, it is obvious that it is a charge which might legitimately be raised on loan, and would cost annually only about £300,000 to the whole United Kingdom.

The annual maintenance and treatment of each patient in the sanatoria might be taken to average £60 to £70 a year, and for 100,000 patients this amounts to six to seven million pounds annually at first; but as time progressed this amount would rapidly drop, and at the end of five or six years would not amount to one million pounds annually.

In casting up the expense of any general scheme to deal with tuberculosis, a certain sum is usually allotted to deal with the upkeep of those from whom the consumptive patient is removed; but very soon when the consumptive is not so removed he becomes unable to work, and then the expense falls inevitably on the public for maintaining his dependents, as it also does on his decease. Hence, except as regards all but a small fraction of the expense, it already has to be publicly borne by the Poor Law Authorities, and when it is considered what a permanent relief from consumptives and their widows and orphans the eradication scheme provides, this charge might still be borne by the local authorities. It would, however borne, be a rapidly decreasing charge.

The only loss of national income would be the wages earned by the one hundred thousand dangerously infective consumptives sent to the sanatoria; and since it is probable that fifty per cent. of these would be incapable of working at all, and the remainder only capable of light intermittent work, and also rapidly passing on to join the incapables, it is clear that the loss on this score would be small, and soon balanced by the thousands saved from infection and remaining sound, fit citizens, capable of good work.

Summing up, then, on this matter of expense, we find that the annual expenditure for consumption eradication would be three hundred thousand for interest on cost of erection of sanatoria to accommodate the patients, and seven millions initially, dropping within five to six years to one million annually, for feeding and attending to the patients. The total amount is less than eight millions a year, even at the outset, and for this sum a disease which now costs the nation at least thirty millions a year can be eradicated with scientific certainty within a period of ten years.

The whole of the burden of the thirty millions would not, of course, drop away during the ten years of eradication, because part of that load is in the form of inherited charges left by departed consumptives. But even within the ten years, the thousands of useful productive lives spared, the decrease in expensive living consumptives, and the commencing decline in number of widows and orphans to be supported, would be more than enough to counterbalance the money directly spent in eradication, and if a careful account of expenditure and saving could be kept for the ten years, the national riches would probably show an increase of several millions.

The cost for tuberculosis eradication would be considerably diminished, and the period for the consummation of effect decreased, if at the same time the National Health Service could be established; but even under our present system, provided a law for compulsory notification and segregation could be brought into action, the disease could be efficiently stamped out.

Without a fairly complete separation of *infective* consumptives, however, no progress of any kind is possible; therein lies the solution of the problem.

The year 1908 is the most recent for which statistics of the United Kingdom can be obtained. That year was the lowest recorded for tuberculosis, and the death-roll for the three kingdoms for tuberculosis of all kinds amounts to somewhat over seventy-four thousand persons; of these deaths, just over fifty-six thousand (56,080) arose from phthisis.

Now, although all of the seventy-four thousand received their illnesses infectively, and our scheme, therefore, will automatically stop all these cases of other forms of tuberculosis, causing eighteen thousand deaths annually, when we stop pulmonary tuberculosis, yet these forms themselves are practically not infective towards healthy people. They arise from smaller numbers of bacilli, buried deep in the bones and elsewhere; there is no sputum containing the infection, and hence we do not need to separate these cases.

This considerably reduces the magnitude of our task, and accordingly we turn to the problem of the isolation of the cases of pulmonary consumption, yielding the 56,080 victims annually.

The first question that arises is whether it is necessary to segregate all the cases giving these fifty-six thousand annual deaths, or if some cases of pulmonary phthisis at certain stages are harmless.

The answer to this question is important, and must be carefully considered in its proper setting. No exceptions must be made which are of danger to the healthy community. No matter what the rank or condition of the victim of pulmonary consumption, care must be taken that he does not sow around, from his infected sputum, the seeds of death in the ways recounted above. There must be one law for rich and poor in this matter; although the burthen on the nation may be somewhat relieved by allowing the patient who can pay to do so, and to be treated in a separate sanatorium under the inspection and control of the State.

The one vital criterion which must be maintained is that *any* patient producing bacilli-laden sputum must live a life apart from the nation in all concerns which may bear infection. He must no longer eat, drink, nor handle, with vessels or implements used in turn by the healthy; he must no longer ride in public conveyances nor go into public buildings; he must eat apart, sleep apart, and work apart from the rest of the community. In exchange, we must provide him with good food, clothing, and residence, in the most healthy surroundings, and attend to his dependents during the period of his separation. *By this procedure, the consumptive himself gains his first real chance of recovery.* He is put, to begin with, under conditions of environment, and a régime of living, which procure him his best chance of recovery. Then, when the disease in his lungs does become arrested, the sputum-producing areas having dried up, and he is now no longer a source of danger, he is turned out into a world cleared of the tubercle bacillus, where it is almost impossible for him to be re-infected and commence again the descent to the valley of the shadow of death. He has, moreover, the satisfaction that he is no longer dragging down with him his wife and family, or others dependent on him, or his co-mates and co-workers in workshop and home.

The next step is to consider the total number of victims of pulmonary disease for whom it would be necessary so to provide.

This figure is an exceedingly difficult one to obtain, because there has hitherto been no compulsory notification of phthisis as there is of most of the acute infectious diseases.

Knowing as we do the number of annual deaths from phthisis, if we could in any way get at the average duration of the dangerous period of a case, then by multiplying these two factors we could obtain the number of dangerous cases co-existing at any given time. For example, did each case last for two years in a dangerous sputum-producing condition, then, with 56,000 deaths annually, there would be $56,000 \times 2 = 112,000$ of such cases at any given time. The average duration, however, is precisely what is so difficult to find out; some cases of pulmonary phthisis last only a few months, while others drag on slowly for many years.

The very slow cases are, however, often so slumbering that little sputum is produced, and many of these cases would probably recover altogether were they not, under our present conditions, reinfected all the time with fresh strains of the infection.

There are accordingly some pulmonary cases which, like the non-pulmonary ones, are almost non-infective, and these, at any rate while the first great strain is on the new system, might be left free. The criterion of freedom should not, however, be the superior surroundings of the patient, more careful nursing, or better education, and better habits of the consumptive. These things are too dangerous in the loopholes they leave to the patient and his friends, and private influences. The State test to be passed by each and every consumptive should be that after a period of observation it is found that he, or she, is either no longer producing any sputum, or a minimal amount which has been carefully examined more than once, and has been passed by a competent bacteriological authority as being at the limit compatible with public safety under definite regulations.

Until the well-to-do consumptive is in this condition he is much better in a sanatorium, both for himself and the public, and when at length he comes forth, if he has conquered in his fight with his enemy, he comes forth into a fresh clean World, where he stands no chance of re-infection. In fact, that country which first puts into operation this system may have to look out within two or three years later for an invasion of wealthy consumptives. The means of guarding from invasion by the disease at our ports will be considered later.

In a book recently published by Latham

and Garland[1] the average duration of phthisis is taken at five years, which gives 280,000 cases of phthisis in the United Kingdom. But in the opinion of the present writer this estimation of duration is too long, and does not make sufficient allowance for the many rapid cases running less than a year.

In any case we have not to deal with the disease from its first inception in the lung until death, and in the author's opinion, after much consideration from many points of view, if we could provide sanatorium accommodation for 100,000 cases, and chose out the 100,000 most dangerous cases all over the Kingdom,[2] we should rapidly break the back of this disease.

It would be unnecessary, with such provision, to allow any dangerously infective case to go free again into the community, and deaths and discharged recoveries would soon make room for the diminishing crops of fresh cases coming in from previously incipient cases. These crops would rapidly decrease in amount, and by the end even of the first year there would be many empty rooms and beds, and

---

[1] "The Conquest of Consumption," by Arthur Latham, M.D., and C. H. Garland (Fisher Unwin, London).

[2] This is the exact reversal of the present rule, which takes incipient and early cases to the sanatoria and turns them out "improved" in three to six months. The present rule is only another example of present-day methods of tinkering the individual case, instead of protecting the community. It is the advanced consumptive who requires to be removed in the community's interests.

in three or four years the sanatoria would gradually empty.

This estimate gives an average period of almost two years of dangerous infectivity for each case of pulmonary phthisis. Taking one case with another, this would probably be ample; a large percentage, especially of the cases first admitted at the commencement, would not last six months, and each such case would allow another chronic case to run three and a half years. Very few cases of a dangerously infective nature would go on for more than three and a half years without either recovery or death.

A system of notification in use in Liverpool during the year 1909, partially voluntary and partially as directed under the Local Government Board Regulations (1908), gave such a number that after deductions of duplicate notifications, other forms of tuberculosis than phthisis, and deaths during the year, the figure remaining (three thousand) bears such a ratio to the number of deaths from phthisis during the year (eleven hundred), that if we take this same ratio for the whole country, where the deaths are 56,000, we reach 153,000 cases as the number of cases which would have been notified during the year and remaining alive at the end of it.

If now we were able to place 100,000 cases in sanatoria, choosing those most dangerous from the public health point of view, there is little doubt that the vast bulk of the dangerously infective cases would be removed from the midst of the community, and the effect of this would soon be obvious. From that time onward the recoveries and deaths in the sanatoria would rapidly make room for cases developing amongst the outside population, and soon the balance would set in the right direction.

In addition to these 100,000 State-provided beds in the national sanatoria, there would be about 5000 private sanatoria beds already in existence throughout the country for paying patients. The enforcement of a law that a consumptive in a condition dangerous to the public health must be removed either to a national or a private sanatorium, and remain there during the continuance of his dangerous condition, would probably lead to the establishment of at least sufficient private paying sanatoria to account for another 10,000 patients.

We come now to the consideration of the question of the compulsory detention of the dangerous consumptive within a sanatorium from the point of view of personal liberty of the individual. We have already seen that it is for the direct advantage of the invalid himself in an undoubted case of phthisis (and we are postulating that the disease is so far advanced that there is sputum being produced, and that this sputum has been shown by a bacteriological examination to contain tubercle bacilli) that he should be so removed and placed under sanatorium conditions. But what are we to do if a silly sentimentality on the part of the patient or his relatives, or both, violently opposes any separation, or insists upon his leaving the sanatorium while still in a dangerous condition for mixing with his friends and the community?

The answer to this question is perfectly clear : the authorities administering the Act must have full powers of removal and detention of all dangerous consumptives, the term "dangerous" being defined as above pointed out.

Nor is there anything novel in such a proposal, for if we remember that phthisis is merely a chronic infectious disease, just as smallpox and scarlet-fever are acute infectious diseases, it will at once be seen that the powers asked in regard to phthisis are merely those supposed by the public to be possessed now by the Public Health Authority in regard to these other infectious diseases.

The Medical Officer of Health of any district, if he is satisfied that any case of a notifiable disease is dangerous to public health, now removes the case to an infectious diseases hospital, and it is detained there until discharge is compatible with public safety.[1]

Only this and nothing more is required in

[1] The Public Health Acts do not really give compulsory powers of removal at present, for these other infectious diseases, and Medical Officers of Health are compelled in the public interests to break the law daily by trading on the patients' ignorance of the law.

the case of phthisis, and, as has already been remarked, if phthisis were not so insidious in its onset, and we could see it strike its victims from one case to another, as we do scarlet-fever and smallpox, we should not still be praying for salvation, but have worked it out long since.

Meanwhile the toll of phthisis is greater than that of all the *acute* infectious diseases put together and added up.

Habit and long custom have made us purblind to the ghastly spectre of consumption stalking about amongst us and casting its invisible darts into the best and cleverest of our citizens, the most beautiful of our women, and the fittest of our men.

This dread disease spares neither the child at school, the athlete in his prime rejoicing in his strength, nor the older man or woman commencing a hale old age ; indiscriminately it attacks all and is no eliminator of the unfit—all, every one amongst us, may be food for it, now or in the future. When shall we wake up?

Although it is essential that the dangerous consumptive shall not mix with the community, there is no reason why he should be entirely cut off from his friends in the matter of visits by them. Each city, or town, or county division would possess its sanatorium, and this might have its weekly visiting day, provided the visitors kept certain isolation rules (the details of which need not be gone into here) intended to safeguard the visitors themselves from infection. To put the matter as briefly as possible, the visitors would have to hold the same attitude towards patients they were visiting as did the members of the medical or nursing staff of the sanatorium, when the risk either of their catching the disease or carrying it out would practically fall to zero.

Another point of great importance, as soon as the system was established, would be the prevention of infection of the country by the arrival of advanced cases of phthisis from foreign ports. Here the risk is much less than with an acutely infectious disease, such as plague or smallpox, yet we know how thoroughly our Port Sanitary Officials are able to protect us from these invasions. Were further proof required of the possibility of guarding our shores from invasion by disease, we have the example of the brilliant achievement of Mr. Walter Long, when Chief of the Local Government Board, in simply annihilating the disease hydrophobia from amongst us, and safeguarding us from re-invasion from abroad.

Previous to the action of Mr. Long, this dread disease was well known in our country, though not so prevalent as in some Continental countries, such as France and Russia. Still, up till then every summer brought Britain its crop of horrible cases of hydrophobia in human beings, and, arising from the hideous character of the disease, its greater crop of terrors from bites of

dogs which might be mad. Since Mr. Walter
Long insisted on efficient action, now about
fourteen years ago, there has not been one single
case of hydrophobia of man or dog throughout
the whole United Kingdom. This fell disease,
still existent in other lands, is extinct in ours.

As we are free now from hydrophobia,
so can we be free from tuberculosis, when
we find a statesman of the courage and
fortitude of Mr. Walter Long to lead us
to victory.

Most of us remember the howls of execration
of the days of the " Muzzling Order " ; it required
some stolidity and grit to stand firm through
that withering fire of criticism and abuse.

Any one who has seen, or even read a detailed
description of the horrors of a case of hydrophobia, can now appreciate what a noble victory was won for us against the votaries of
sentimentality in those days ; and not the least
thankful, if they could understand and speak,
would be the dogs themselves. Not only have
all British dogs escaped hydrophobia ; hundreds
of them have escaped being shot or stoned to
death by frenzied and infuriated mobs, madder
than the supposed mad dogs they engaged in
hounding to death.

The fundamental quarantine rules against
phthisis are quite obvious, especially as it is the
more advanced cases which are the real danger.
Every case of immigration suspected of phthisis
—and the disease at a stage when dangerous to

others usually holds out plain enough signals —must be examined. When the lesions of phthisis are found present, admission to the country must be refused, and this rule must suffer no violation.

The chief steamship lines, once they knew that phthisical patients would be returned on their hands, would soon set up medical examinations and cease booking them, and the number of cases requiring to be submitted to careful or prolonged examination at our ports of entry from abroad would soon diminish to a small percentage of the total arrivals.

M

CHAPTER VI

THE EVOLUTION OF THE NATIONAL MEDICAL SERVICE

A RETROSPECT over the preceding chapters, which have been chiefly concerned in pointing out evils and abuses, produces rather the impression of blackness and darkness than that of any approach to dawn. Still, the darkest hour is that before the dawn, the horizon is even now just commencing to show the light of approaching day, and certain glad notes of song proclaim that every one is not asleep to the breath of morning.

The sunrise that is coming will not be a tropical outburst suddenly dazzling the World and flooding it with light, but will come with the ever-increasing glory of a morning in temperate climes. At first, but the grey of dawn in the East, showing how black the darkness has been ; then, golden-hued clouds with a background of many-tinted haze, increasing in radiance and beauty of colouring as the Sun approaches, followed by the grand outburst as the god of day comes in sight.

It is by a process of organic evolution, and not by any creative act of a single mind, that

the health era will be established.   Always in
evolutionary processes it is observable that the
first movements are slow and apparently un-
certain in their purpose, but as the process
advances the rate of progress ever quickens.

The social world has not been still during
the past fifty years in matters of hygiene and
public health ; bad as things are to-day, and
little as we should be satisfied with them,
they were much worse a generation ago.

But just now there is a great and general
awakening of the public mind, voiced by the
thoughts and actions of millions of the best of
the inhabitants of the country, towards a real
scientific and continued endeavour to deal with
the problems of poverty and disease in a way
that means eradication from the race, and
not merely amelioration of the lot of the
individual.

Philanthropy in the true sense, based on
scientific forethought, is taking the place of
soft-headed and soft-hearted charity.   Instead
of giving away of our surplus riches to the
poor, in soul-destroying doles, we are commencing to realise that we must give instead
some of our surplus brains to the understand-
ing of this problem, which is our problem as
well as the poor man's problem, and that we
must better the position of the poor in spite
of the things which we have previously been
content to call their vices.   These people have
neither the intellect nor the moral stamina to

get rid of these vices without help, and the very vices are the result of these defects of theirs, and not of any intentional human perversity planted in them by the Creator of the Universe. These poor creatures represent the so-called survival of the fittest in a perverted environment, and show the best that an unaided environment can do: it is ours to better that environment, and bring forth a fitter race for humanity's high purposes, just as we have done in the culture of the Earth, and of the lower creation. We who can see thus far, have a mission in evolution, and a command to go forth and make the World somewhat better because we have lived in it, both for our own generation and for those to follow, of which we are to be the progenitors and leaders. It matters not that we do not understand the whole of the riddle; let us follow what we know to be our best instincts, and in the unravelling during our lives of a little of the great puzzle we can have our greatest pleasure and happiest life. Who can tell but one day we shall see the whole, and with added pleasure because we have borne a share in producing the beauty of it all!

The construction of a National Health Service to produce the good fruits in strengthening the physique of the race, and saving the national resources as outlined in the previous chapters, is a process which will require a generation for its completion, and the collaboration of many active minds of skilful administrators.

Accordingly, but little service would be done by attempting a detailed forecast of the operations of such a service completely equipped and in full working order. Any such scheme could be quickly torn to pieces by the destructive criticism of those who always see impossibilities in difficulties, and believe that "whatever is, is best."

The first essential towards reform is to show the existence of evil in present methods, and when that has been done all that is good in our human nature will go on patiently testing one experience after another towards the removal of the evil.

Any constructive details which may appear in the sketch about to be given of the path of evolution of the National Medical Service of the future, are put forward quite tentatively, and to a great extent as material for discussion, for the elaboration of a plan of work which must inevitably suffer infinite variation as reform progresses and new measures are required to meet new situations which have arisen by the way.

With these reservations, some attempt may now be made to sketch the path along which the evolution of a National Health Service, specially designed for disease prevention and elimination, will probably come to us.

There are two great movements in present-day politics, supported in principle by both of the great political parties, which must ere long find their expression in legislation, and such legislation, if conceived in any true sense on National lines, must inevitably lead to the establishment sooner or later of one unified and co-ordinated National Medical Service.

The two movements referred to are (1) the provision of a National System of Insurance against Sickness, and (2) the Reform of the Poor Law as advocated by the Reports of the Royal Commission. In reality these two movements, arising in quite different ways, are bound sooner or later to converge into a common scheme which will supply medical attendance and treatment to the whole of the wage-earning classes—that is to say, to about thirty-eight millions of people in these countries.

Economics demand that such a service, soon after its complete establishment, shall become preventive in its mode of action.

The most ardent section of Poor Law reformers—namely, those who uphold the Minority Report—advocate the establishment of a unified system of County Medical Services in which the Public Health Services and Poor Law Services shall become amalgamated under the various municipalities, other services than those connected with sickness of the present Poor Law Guardians passing to various discrete existent bodies. The weakness of this otherwise admirable policy lies in the inadequate co-ordination of the municipalities with one another which we already experience in the case of the present Poor Law Unions. When the system becomes established, as it probably soon will be with minor alterations, this weakness will become apparent, and either all these many Municipal Health Authorities will be thrown into one National Service, or a very strong Central Body (much stronger than anything postulated in the Minority Report) will be formed, controlling and correlating these services and substantially uniting them in a way which that body, with so multifarious duties, called the Local Government Board, is supposed to do for the present Poor Law Service, but so signally fails to do.

One great defect of a system consisting of a large number of Municipal Services, as compared with a National Service, is the impossibility of affording adequate opportunities for merit to show itself in the Service all over the country.

A man cannot, within the boundaries of the same service, be transferred and promoted from one local centre to another as he can under a National Service; nor can the local services acquire sufficient strength and wealth in most cases, excepting in very large cities, to provide post-graduate training colleges and hospitals such as are provided now, for example, by the medical services of our Army and Navy, for keeping members of the Medical Staff up-to-date with their work, and giving them periods of recuperation and revival at stated intervals.

There are other defects inherent in local machinery, especially in regard to medical matters, such, for example, as want of medical knowledge on the part of local laymen of supervision of medical work, wire-pulling over local appointments, sweating of salaries or its reverse, and other such things, which need not here be elaborated at length.

For these reasons, it is probable that the unified County Medical Services will only be a valuable temporary measure towards a final National Medical Service, as far as Poor Law medical work is concerned.

Of greater magnitude, since it concerns many times more people, and carries in its train much more deeply seated changes, is the National Sickness Insurance Scheme, which also leads, though by a longer path, to a National Medical Service in the end.

Here there stand, at the outset, two great vested interests, like two lions in the path, each opposed to and unfriendly with the other, and both more or less opposed, chiefly on account of ignorance, to the National Scheme.

There is no room for the National Insurance Scheme to exist along with these two irreconcilable interests. Without confiscation or spoliation, and with all equity, it must, if it is to be a success, simply swallow both of them up by a process of absorption and assimilation.

These two great vested interests are (1) The Friendly Societies, (2) The Medical Profession, and in both cases the people concerned must be made, without detriment to themselves, part and parcel of the National Sickness Insurance Scheme.

Considering first the Friendly Societies, it is obvious, as the chief officials of the big societies have already realised, that setting up a great National Society in rivalry to them, able to enforce subsidies from the employers, would simply ruin them. They would in the end be equally, though more slowly, ruined if the Government gave them equal privileges with itself, and there would arise, in addition, the trouble and expense of distributing the employers' quota of the subscriptions to the many Friendly Societies.

But it would be suicidal to the National Scheme, and at the same time an unwarrantable increasing of vested interests which would be almost impossible to get rid of afterwards, to expand the present Friendly Societies to at least six times their present size so that they looked after the Sickness Insurance of all the workers.

Such a colossal folly as this would outmagnify such things as Telephone leases a hundred-fold, and establish a monopoly more powerful than "The Trade," so it is to be hoped that whatever statesman, or political party, finally carries through State Sickness Insurance will have strength and stability enough to remain unmoved by the supposed vote-casting powers of the members of the Friendly Societies.[1]

Since the present staffs of the Friendly Societies only carry out the secretarial and organising work of the insurance of about one-sixth of the numbers to be insured under any National Insurance Scheme, it is obvious that work can be found for all of them in the offices of the National Insurance Bureau directed by the Minister of Public Health. The funds and properties of the Societies can be similarly dealt with, the sum to which each member is entitled being dealt with in one of three ways :—(1) It can be returned to him in cash; (2) it can be invested for him in Government Securities; (3) it can be written down to him as so much surplus Sickness Insurance money above the minimum required by the State Insurance Act, or used for a definite length of time in paying off his own contribution towards his insurance.

The action of the United States Government in regard to the affairs of one great Insurance

---

[1] The German State Insurance Scheme has almost suffered shipwreck, because administration was left largely in the hands of the German Friendly Societies. Even now, the German doctors in many parts of that country are deeply dissatisfied with it, and are in almost open revolt against it, on account of antipathy to the methods of the Friendly Societies. No true service can be obtained under sweating conditions, and this is what we shall have unless our new State Sickness Insurance is run on National lines, and without the embarrassment of hundreds of competing Societies, providing salaries for unnecessary middlemen.

Company shows that the Government of any country has a perfectly equitable right to interfere in the affairs of any public company in such a fashion.

Moreover, there is little question that the present members of Friendly Societies, if consulted, would agree by large majorities to be transferred to the National Scheme, under some such equitable conditions as have been outlined above.[1]

The solution of the difficulty created by the existence of the numerous Friendly Societies accordingly lies not in granting new powers or extensions to these, nor in setting up anything in rivalry to them, but purely in *absorbing* them with absolute justice to both officials and members. If a strong statesman puts forward a sound National Scheme, the absorption will not prove a process of any great difficulty.

Gradual absorption is also the natural process in the case of the other great vested interest involved, namely, that of the medical profession.

----

[1] According to the returns of the Chief Registrar of Friendly Societies, the aggregate membership of "Ordinary Friendly Societies" is 3,473,712, and of Friendly Societies with branches (such as Foresters and Oddfellows) the total membership is 2,704,404. This means only about one-sixth of the population to be insured, and of these there is no doubt that the majority would support any equitable Government Scheme for absorption, whatever officials may say. The members have joined these Societies because no Government Scheme has existed, and the endowment of a properly constituted National System would remove entirely the *raison d'être* of these Societies, a fact which their own members will be the first to realise.

If this vested interest did not exist, the National Medical Service would undoubtedly be manned from the beginning by a Staff paid by salary for whole-time service, and towards this the constant movement ought to be directed. To turn the whole of the present medical men practising in the country immediately into salaried medical officers would, however, prove impossible. There exists no basis, to begin with, upon which the salaries of the doctors could be calculated in a trustworthy way, and such a basis must first be obtained.

For the first period of running of the scheme, then, it would have to be thrown open to the whole of the medical profession, and payment would have to be made upon the basis of some scheme such as one or other of several plans, differing in detail, which have been discussed by the British Medical Association and other bodies.

This arrangement, however, does not preclude working towards the ideal of a true National Medical Service with proper admissions, and promotions, and opportunities for service and study. In fact, the gradual evolution of a service such as can be brought about in the course of at most twenty to twenty-five years, without any sudden or revolutionary procedures, will only tend to the organic development of a much better service.

After the State Insurance Scheme had run for a period of, say, three years, there are two methods by which it could be gradually converted into a National Medical Service.

As soon as the State Insurance came into action, a State Examination should be established for entry into the State Medical Service,[1] and during the first three years the entrants into the State service should be sent into the State hospitals which the new scheme would inevitably require. The number of men required each year in this way would be 800 to 1000, for there are about 32,000 members of the medical profession, and assigning thirty-five years of active life service to each man, the annual number required for maintenance of the staff of the service would be thus about nine hundred men.[2]

At the end of the three preliminary years, a basis would have been obtained on which incomes could be calculated, and then inducements of a steady income, based on these figures in each case, with such retirement allowances as every medical man ought to have at the age of sixty-five, should be offered, in order to induce men in practice to become members of the National Medical Service.

The places of men retiring, and the vacancies

---

[1] In a few years this State Examination would become a single portal entry to the medical profession, that great desideratum of many years which has never yet been realised.

[2] These new State hospitals and State doctors do not mean additional expense, for, as has previously been shown, we have already to pay for both hospitals and doctors in many devious and most uneconomical ways.

left by deaths of practitioners, would be filled by drafting in the men who had meanwhile been undergoing training in the State hospitals.

There is little doubt that at the end of the three years a large number of existing practitioners would choose to join the State Medical Service.[1]

Even without any such adhesions, in a period of about twenty-five years the State Service would automatically have established itself, and in the best possible way, namely, that of slow organic growth.

With such a service in operation, and the numerous State hospitals in connection with it carrying out efficient medical and surgical work, and the State Medical Staff coming in, by rotation, to acquire hospital skill, it would soon be found that the Voluntary Hospitals would step into line with the rest of the service and accept State support and control.

The final result would be one unified system in common co-ordination of hospitals and doctors, now no longer in deadly opposition to one another, but working for a common cause—in short, a modern machine and weapon of warfare against disease, instead of a fragmentary and motley museum of survivals from antiquity.

Now let us glance at this machine at work.

---

[1] In a referendum now being taken of all Medical men in Ireland, 1765 have voted For, and only 35 Against, the institution of a National Medical Service for Ireland.

The district assigned to each State doctor
doing outside work would contain 400 to 500
families or houses.[1]   He would have in this
district a surgery to which any one requiring
advice would come at fixed times of consultation; there would be no crowds, as at present,
because there would be no sweated work; there
would be no advanced phthisical cases coming,
because they, if still existent, would be in sanatoria; other infectious cases would also be
chiefly picked out in the homes, in ways to
be pointed out later.   Such patients who came
on their own initiative would be treated in
the surgery as at present, but on account of
other agencies at work the number would be
much less than at present.   No case of serious
disease would be allowed to go away treated
in a perfunctory way, or sent back into the
community or to work.   The infectious case
would go to the infectious hospital, or if circumstances were such that it could be isolated,
and rendered free of danger to others, it would
be treated at home.   Similarly, with the serious
case, such as one requiring a surgical operation,
this would be sent to the hospital, or if the
patient refused he would be told flatly and
straightforwardly the great risk he was running;

[1] This would constitute each doctor's district for inspection
and preventive purposes, but for the purpose of patients visiting doctors for advice on their own initiative, a dozen or more
such districts might be termed a division, within which any
patient might make choice of a doctor without having to pay
a fee, so preserving the choice of doctor.

there would be no hospital abuse existing any longer, and no fees at stake. The effect of such things as these in diminishing the flow of disease through the doctors' surgeries can be imagined.

Then at certain hours the doctor would do his visiting rounds much as he does at present, but under much more ideal conditions than he can now claim. He would have no rivals worrying him, no bills to bother about, no suspicions lest his patients thought he was after fees. His practice would be compact in the little district allotted to him, and while there would be sufficient supervision to see there was no shirking of work, he would be free from a hundred embarrassments in his work from which he now suffers.

Let us next look at the matter from the point of view, so often called in evidence by opponents, of "the Sanctity of the Home" and the intrusion upon it of an army of officials.

This is an ancient bogey which was taken out of its cupboard, carefully dusted, and filled with fresh straw, to alarm the British workman and voter when free education was granted him for his children.

He was then told that his hereditary castle was gone for ever, and that he would have no peace or quiet with his wife and family on account of the unwelcome and prying visits of the School Attendance Officer haling poor little Johnnie away to school as to some prison or torture chamber.

Now is it so in fact, after a good many years of reign of the School Board? Is this reign really a reign of terror? Is the School Attendance Officer an irksome person in constant attendance at the poor man's house? No; he is only a terror to those, and they are but a small percentage, to whom he ought to be a terror, and to whom we would all wish him to be a terror, who neglect their children in a wicked and criminal way.

Similarly with the Sanitary Inspector of Nuisances, and the inspectors for cruelty and neglect of children. These officials, although they visit homes, have no more terrors for honest people than either the policeman or the gas-meter inspector.

There is also that utterly uncalled-for figment of the imagination of a frequent inspection of the healthy to be dealt with. No such compulsory inspection of healthy people is necessary in tracking down and beating out disease. If we have an efficient National Health Corps whose business it is to find infectious disease and stamp it out, the object can be achieved without any vexatious examination or interference with the healthy. All this is no refutation of what has been said previously that it is a sane and sensible thing for a person to be examined once a year whether he is feeling ill or not, just as it is a wise

N

thing to let a dentist look at the teeth occasionally. But no one need be compelled to do it who does not want to do so.

Let us see how the National Medical Service would get its work of prevention in. Suppose a case of diphtheria has been found in a given house in a given street. Then, first of all, that case, unless it could be properly isolated and treated in the house, would be *at once* removed and treated with antitoxin at the Infectious Diseases Hospital, without any waiting, or any orders, or other nonsensical preliminaries, with the result that the life would often be saved where it is now lost. An intimation would, of course, be sent to the school the patient had been attending, and to all the doctors in neighbouring districts who were responsible for the patient's classmates, and the school medical officer's task would be to catch the first sore throat turning up in that school, send the child home, and have it watched by its own district medical officer.

The duty of the district medical officer who first found the case would be to question the mother as to the people who had been in contact with the child, keep these under observation, and make inquiries either himself or through the district nurse, or by any voluntary health-workers attached to his district, as to sore throats in these houses. A simple inquiry at the door is all that is required: " Anybody in the house suffering from cold or sore throat?" An affirmative answer would bring the doctor to examine into the matter. Is there anything inquisitorial in such methods, or does any one think it would be resented by people who know they are paying for the doctor, and for just such care being exercised for them? If there are people so ignorant as to resent such things, then the sooner we educate them otherwise, and teach them it is a privilege to be cared for, the better.

In addition to this, it ought to be the district doctor's business, or that of one of his Staff, to call at least once in six months and simply ask if all is well in a household; there need be no inquisition and no forcible entry. Some educative teaching as to the value of early acquainting the doctor with cases of illness, given with the object-lesson of a neglected case, would soon do away with any tendency to conceal illness in the household, and the National Medical Service would soon acquire the confidence of the people. The absence of the dread of the fee to pay amongst the poor, or rather the comforting thought that it had already been paid in the weekly contribution, would also tend to create ready confidence between doctor and patient. The lay officials of the Government would assist the doctor in combating any dishonest malingering, another bogey about which far too much fuss is made. Soon this house-to-house visiting, and reminding people that they had the services of a doctor at their call, would become unnecessary as they became educated up to the new order of things. Disease would reach the doctor earlier, and the outlook would improve both for patient and community. Under such conditions the Public Health would unquestionably so much improve, and widespread epidemics of disease become so rare, that more and more of the time of the medical staff would become free from tinkering of patients, and capable of utilisation for direct attack upon disease and its prevention, and for inquiry and research upon the problems of health and disease.

One note which cannot be too often repeated is that such a service would not tend in the least to the protection of the unfit, but on the contrary, by producing a more and more healthy environment, would develop a more and more healthy species to inhabit that environment. Do not let us, by a false application of the law of the survival of the fittest, fall a-slumbering to the fact that even the fittest for a wretched environment may not be the finest race. The misapplication of this fundamental biological law is one of the greatest delusions of the superficial knowledge of the age, a product of that half-knowledge which is so intensely dangerous.

Let us improve the environment, and the wretched creatures of the environment will improve with it and grow into the fittest for the new and better environment we have provided.

Also, do not let us think the less fit will over-run the earth if they be helped up. Nature herself looks after that; the exact opposite is the truth—they will over-run the earth if they are not raised up. If the bad environment is made the almost universal one, as it is now, the lower type of creature in that environment will over-run the higher type. We are one species, we human-kind, and one class cannot safely or permanently rise or fall by itself; we must take the others up, or be dragged down ourselves along with them.

APPENDIX

THE second supplement to the last decennial report of the Registrar-General of Births, Deaths, and Marriages (Blue Book, published 1908) contains a detailed account of occupational mortality amongst males, in which the figures for total deaths, due to several important diseases, in each of 104 classes of occupations, are given for the years 1900–1902. The ratio of deaths from phthisis to total deaths, in various occupations, shows in a most interesting manner how the death-rate rises in those occupations where the workmen are more subjected to close contact with their fellows, *at the later and more infectious stages of the disease.* It is not dust-laden atmosphere or confined space which increase the death-rate from phthisis, so much as the presence in close proximity of phthisical fellow-workmen in the infective stages of the disease. In support of this the various occupations are arranged in the table given below in order of the ratio of the phthisis-deaths to total-deaths from all causes.

The following remarks regarding certain typical employments may illustrate the value of the tabulation.

One of the heaviest death-rates of all is amongst printers, compositors, and lithographers, where nearly one in every three dies of phthisis. Here we have an occupation in which a workman can go on with his work to the very end, and where he is working close to other workmen, and using the same tools, at a stage when he is most highly infective. The author has recently had considerable opportunity, on account of intimate business relationships with compositors, of studying this problem, and discussing it with some of those intimately concerned. The workmen do not appear to realise how insidiously infective this disease is, and blame the dust and closeness of their occupation as the cause of the excessive death-rate. This is not the true cause ; coal-miners, who work in most confined spaces and have most dusty work, have a death-rate from phthisis of only about one in eleven. The coal-miner who contracts phthisis somewhere else than at his work, has to leave off his heavy physical labours before he reaches the advanced stage at which he becomes dangerous to his fellow-workers. Also, he does not work

199

in such close companionship with them, and at intervals use the same tools and appliances. It appears that in any large compositors' workroom there is usually to be found at least one individual with more or less advanced phthisis, who uses the same tools, the same towels for washing up, and so on, as all the other workmen. It would pay the healthy workmen out of their society funds to retire such men altogether, rather than be saddled with a death-rate of one in three from the operation of such obvious causes.

The same thing is illustrated by the low phthisis death-rate amongst marine firemen and stokers. Here the confined sleeping accommodation, the vicissitudes of temperature on and off work, the coal-dust, and so on, would have been factors inclining one *prima facie* to place stokers near the head of the list; but, strange to say, they have a death-rate from phthisis of only one in eleven. The explanation is that they do not infect one another. Before the disease has advanced to its infective stage the stoker is no longer fit for his work.

Other influences undoubtedly come in, such as open-air life and good food, or the reverse of these, as is shown by the ten occupations at the end of the list, but a glance at the occupations at the upper end of the list (all those up to 5·5, for example, except dock-labourers) shows in a convincing way that these are as a rule light occupations in which the consumptive can stay at work and go on infecting his fellow-workmen long after he has reached the infective stage of the disease.

The contrast between dock-labourers with an incidence of two in eleven, and navvies and road-labourers with about one in twelve, or bargemen and lightermen with two in twenty-five, is remarkable. It indicates the dreadful effects of casual labour, underfeeding, and overcrowding in the houses, as an object-lesson to which it would be hard to find an equal.

The whole list is of intense value as an indication, under present conditions, of those employments which the threatened consumptive, or person of weak physique, should avoid, and of those which offer a better chance of safety.

The variation in incidence from one in three, to one in twenty-seven, shows the enormous influence of occupation, education, and environment. It may be pointed out that the excessively low rate amongst clergymen is not due to the extremely good health of clergymen on the whole; because it is a ratio of deaths from phthisis to deaths from all causes, and, therefore, although clergymen have the healthiest lives in the community, this does not explain the low phthisical death-ratio. For, as a result of the low general death-rate, both phthisis death-rate and general death-rate would go down together, and so the ratio would remain undisturbed. Accordingly the ratio of one in twenty-seven amongst clergymen demonstrates something more than this. It clearly shows that phthisis is a disease due mainly to ignorance, carelessness, and infection under dirty surroundings, and that we can get rid of it effectually when we are prepared to organise and fight against it.

It is a high honour to the clergy that they possess not only the lowest general death-rate in the country, but comparatively, on the top of this, the very lowest death-ratio from phthisis. Such figures indicate for the profession the highest standard of pure, clean, healthy living in the whole country. Is it too much to appeal to this highest rank of teachers in the nation, who are themselves setting such a noble example, to recognise that the highest ideals of their religion demand a crusade to make their own death-rate from phthisis the death-rate of the nation. It is not necessary that the country should be oppressed and impoverished by our present incidences of illness ; the cause of our afflictions is our apathy and carelessness of all that science has taught.

OCCUPATIONAL DEATH-RATES FROM PHTHISIS AND FROM ALL CAUSES RESPECTIVELY, AND THE RATIO OF PHTHISIS DEATH-RATE TO TOTAL DEATH-RATE.

(For all males over 15 years of age, whether occupied or retired,[1] in England and Wales only, during three years 1900–1902.)

OCCUPATION (All Occupations)	TOTAL DEATHS FROM PHTHISIS (66,937)	TOTAL DEATHS FROM ALL CAUSES (509,567)	RATIO (7·6)
Inn and Hotel Servants .	646	2,109	1 death in 3·3
Printers	946	3,209	,, 3·4
Tramway Service Employees . . .	131	494	,, 3·8
Commercial Clerks . .	2,422	9,807	., 4·0
Law Clerks	235	956	,, 4·1
Bookbinders . . .	120	490	,, 4·1
Hairdressers . . .	270	1,183	,, 4·4
Musicians	247	1,143	,, 4·6
Railway Clerks and Officials	420	2,079	,, 4·9

[1] The incidence amongst the employed only is still higher than that amongst employed and retired counted together, because the incidence of phthisis is higher in middle life.

OCCUPATION (All Occupations)	TOTAL DEATHS FROM PHTHISIS (66,937)	TOTAL DEATHS FROM ALL CAUSES (509,567)	RATIO (7·6)
Tobacconists . . .	156	784	1 death in 5·0
Drapers, etc. . . .	469	2,399	,, 5·1
Tool, Scissor, File Makers .	490	2,519	,, 5·1
Glass Manufacturers . .	223	1,135	,, 5·1
Messengers and Porters (not Rly. or Gvt.) . . .	833	4,344	,, 5·2
Hatters	156	812	,, 5·2
India-rubber, Gutta, etc., Workers	81	419	,, 5·2
Domestic Indoor Servants .	329	1,781	,, 5·4
Costermongers, Hawkers .	833	4,492	,, 5·4
Dock Labourers . . .	1,036	5,709	,, 5·5
Watch and Clock Makers, Jewellers, etc. . .	626	3,463	,, 5·5
Copper, Tin, Zinc, Lead, Brass, etc., Workers .	1,138	6,357	,, 5·6
Cabinetmakers, etc. . .	775	4,383	,, 5·7
Stationers, Publishers, Newsagents . . .	379	2,148	,, 5·7
Potters, Earthenware Workers, etc. . . .	306	1,770	,, 5·8
Civil Service (Messengers)	264	1,553	,, 5·9
Brush, Brooms, Hair, Bristle Workers	102	601	,, 5·9
Paperhangers, Plasterers, etc.	318	1,909	,, 6·0
Plumbers, Painters, Glaziers	1,605	9,751	,, 6·1
Coach, Cab, Omnibus Service, Grooms . . .	1,641	10,248	,, 6·2
Boiler-makers, Fitters, Millwrights, etc. . . .	1,963	12,164	,, 6·2
Stone and Slate Quarries .	504	3,141	,, 6·2
Saddlers, Harness Makers .	206	1,298	,, 6·3
Schoolmasters . . .	280	1,781	,, 6·4
Shoemakers . . .	1,886	12,027	,, 6·4
Curriers	182	1,169	,, 6·4
Tailors	1,171	7,658	,, 6·5
Wood-turners, Coopers, etc.	312	2,035	,, 6·5
Cotton Manufacturers .	1,157	7,497	,, 6·5
Lace Manufacturers . .	87	567	,, 6·5

OCCUPATION (All Occupations)	TOTAL DEATHS FROM PHTHISIS (66,937)	TOTAL DEATHS FROM ALL CAUSES (509,567)	RATIO (7·6)
Bricklayers, Masons, etc. . .	2,521	16,632	1 death in 6·6
Coal-heavers . . .	204	1,356	,, 6·6
General Shopkeepers . .	273	1,852	,, 6·8
Paper Manufacturers . .	70	474	,, 6·8
Chimney Sweeps . .	80	543	,, 6·8
Commercial Travellers .	419	2,880	,, 6·9
Ironmongers . . .	125	887	,, 7·1
Carmen and Carriers . .	1,499	10,789	,, 7·2
Brewers . . .	244	1,749	,, 7·2
Slaters, Tilers . .	65	467	,, 7·2
General Labourers . .	7,197	52,004	,, 7·2
Railway Guards, Porters, Pointsmen . .	604	4,439	,, 7·3
Bakers, Confectioners .	550	4,036	,, 7·3
Dyers (Textile) . .	324	2,407	,, 7·4
Gas Workers . .	262	1,979	,, 7·5
AVERAGE	66,937	509,567	,, 7·6
All Textiles . . .	2,313	17,788	,, 7·7
Fishmongers, Poulterers .	164	1,278	,, 7·8
Grocers, etc. . .	647	5,045	,, 7·8
Artists, Sculptors, Architects	127	1,003	,, 7·9
Railway Engine Drivers and Stokers . . .	185	1,475	,, 7·9
Nail, Anchor, Chain, etc., Makers . . .	1,364	10,774	,, 7·9
Seamen (Merchant Service)	1,006	8,128	,, 8·1
Butchers . . .	569	4,675	,, 8·2
Coach, Carriage, etc., Makers	237	1,937	,, 8·2
Chemists and Druggists .	142	1,281	,, 8·3
Civil Service (Officers and Clerks) . . .	253	2,138	,, 8·4
Fruiterers, Greengrocers .	223	1,882	,, 8·4
Carpenters, Joiners . .	1,398	11,924	,, 8·5
Carpet, Felt, etc., Workers	46	415	,, 9·0
Shipbuilders . .	388	3,607	,, 9·3
Wool, etc., Manufacturers .	474	4,393	,, 9·3
Blacksmiths, Strikers, etc. .	718	6,972	,, 9·7
Rope, Twine, etc., Manufacturers . . .	43	440	,, 10·2

OCCUPATION (All Occupations)	TOTAL DEATHS FROM PHTHISIS (66,937)	TOTAL DEATHS FROM ALL CAUSES (509,567)	RATIO (7·6)
Innkeepers, Publicans .	933	9,608	1 death in 10·3
All Miners	2,253	23,190	,, 10·3
Sawyers . . .	147	1,570	,, 10·7
Brick, Tile, etc., Makers .	166	1,820	,, 10·9
Hosiers	106	1,165	,, 11·0
Coal Miners . . .	1,950	21,605	,, 11·1
Wheelwrights . . .	140	1,574	,, 11·2
Firemen, Stokers, Marine Engineers . . .	371	4,136	,, 11·2
Maltsters	40	466	,, 11·6
Millers, etc. . . .	113	1,306	,, 11·6
Silk, etc., Manufacturers .	76	904	,, 11·8
Platelayers, Rly. Labourers, Navvies, Road Labourers	629	7,471	,, 11·9
Milksellers, Cheesemongers	167	2,022	,, 12·1
Chemical Manufacturers .	86	1,055	,, 12·3
Bargemen and Lightermen.	174	2,170	,, 12·5
Gardeners, Nurserymen .	669	9,674	,, 14·5
Coal Merchants and Dealers	121	1,780	,, 14·7
Barristers and Solicitors .	80	1,181	,, 14·8
Fishermen	85	1,347	,, 15·8
Farm Labourers . . .	1,679	28,745	,, 17·1
Gamekeepers . . .	46	829	,, 18·0
Farmers and Graziers .	884	19,447	,, 22·0
Physicians	59	1,342	,, 22·7
Clergymen	92	2,488	,, 27·0

Printed by BALLANTYNE, HANSON & Co.
Edinburgh & London

CPSIA information can be obtained
at www.ICGtesting.com
Printed in the USA
LVHW081644250421
685527LV00004B/128

9 781378 924327